THIS PLANNER BELONGS TO

_____

Contact:

_____

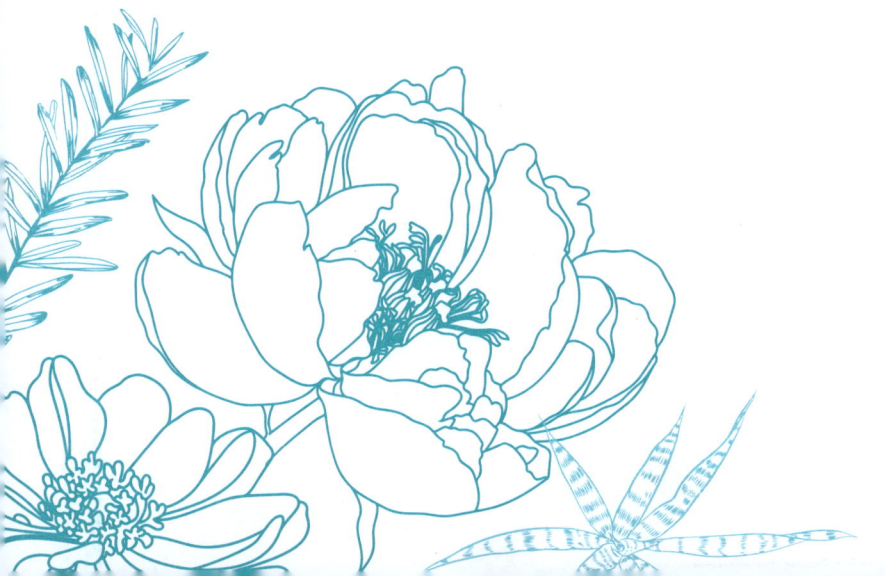

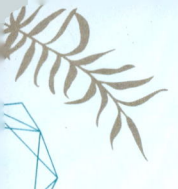

BIRTHDAYS & DATES TO REMEMBER

Birthdays *Dates to Remember*

DATE	WHO	DATE	EVENT

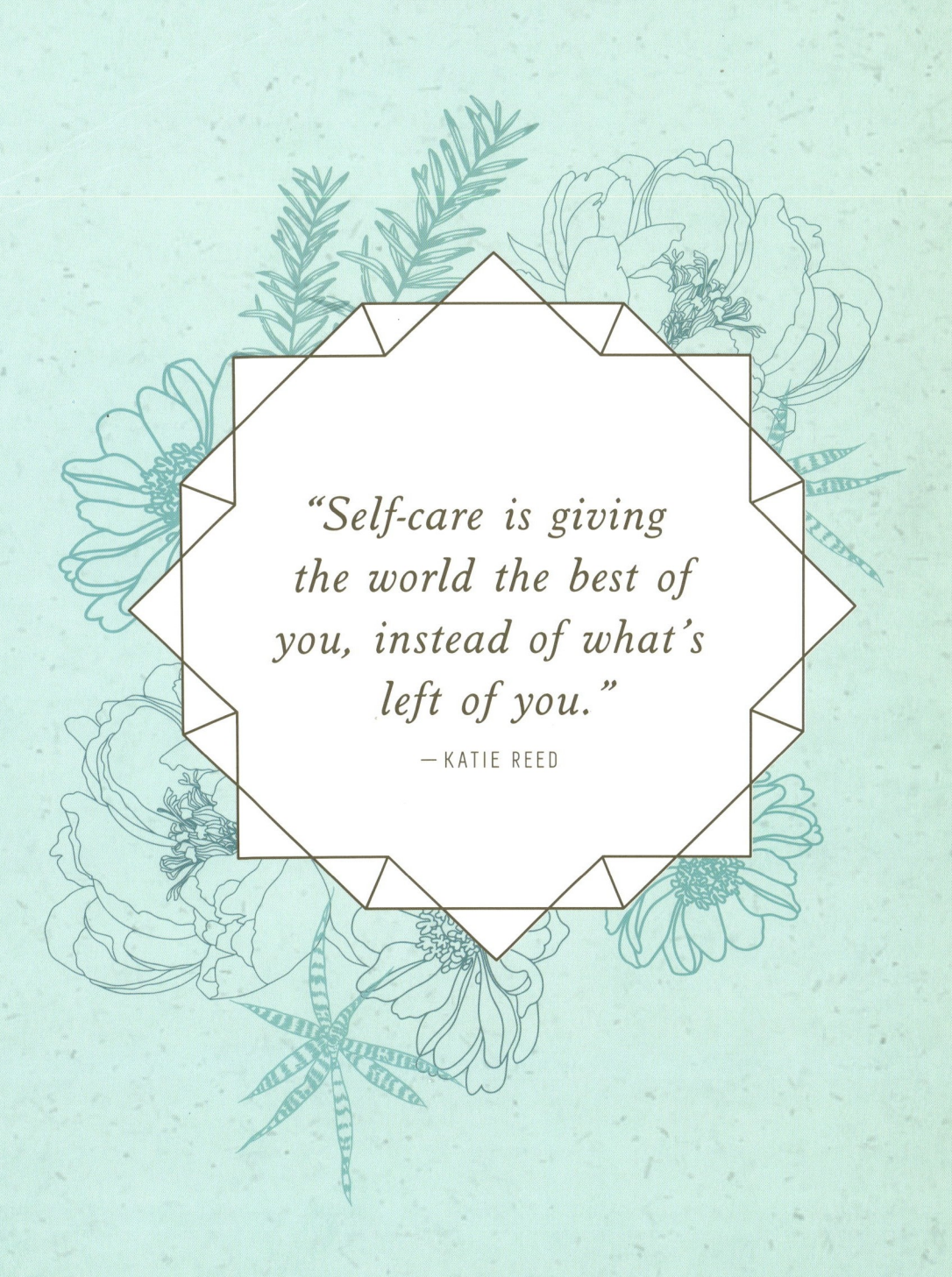

"Self-care is giving the world the best of you, instead of what's left of you."

— KATIE REED

SELF-CARE
priorities

SELF-CARE
IS NOT SELFISH.
YOU CANNOT
SERVE FROM AN
EMPTY VESSEL.
—Eleanor Brownn

Monday	*Tuesday*	*Wednesday*

NOTES

Thursday	Friday	Saturday	Sunday

BIRTHDAYS

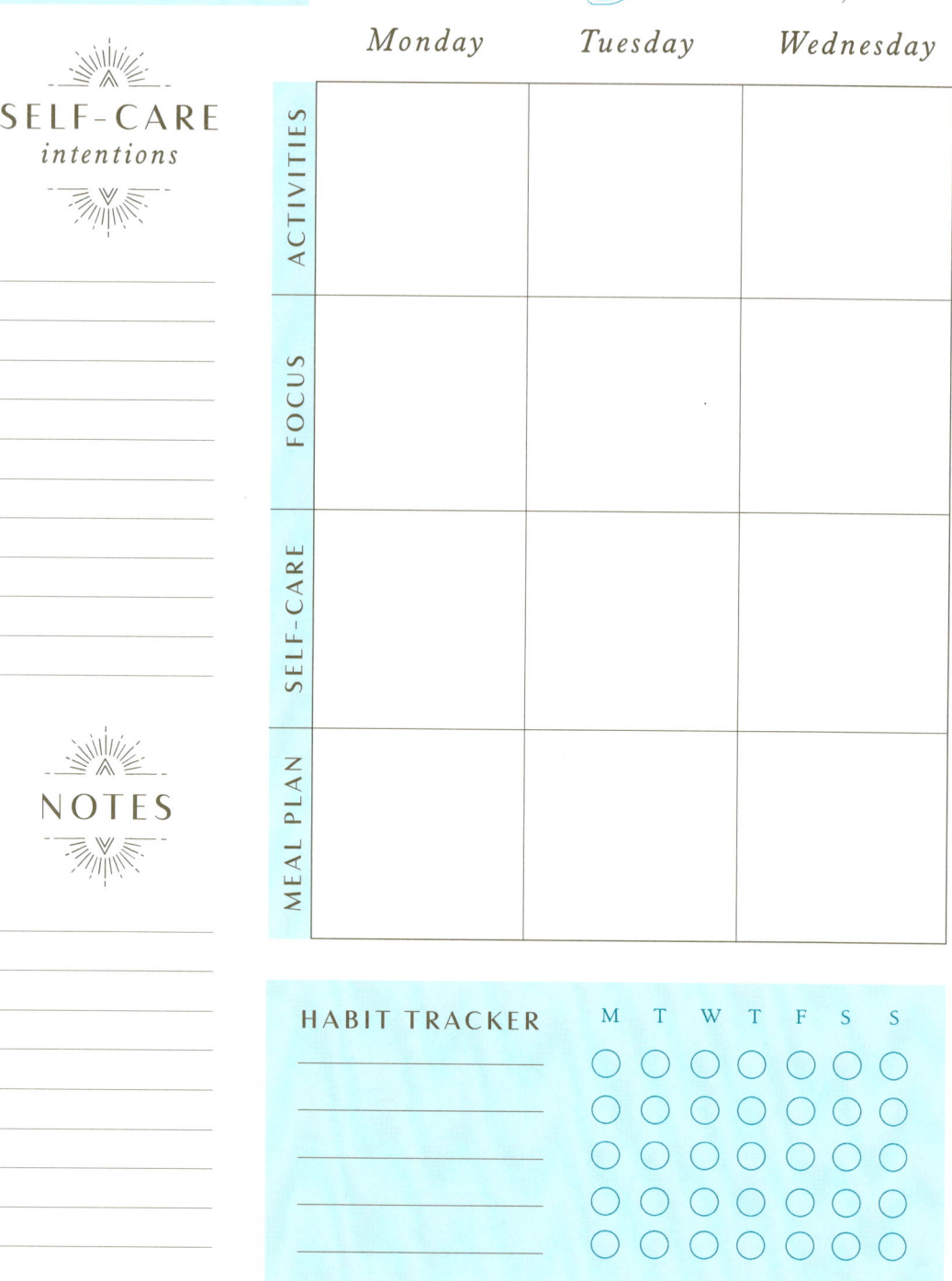

Thursday	*Friday*	*Saturday*	*Sunday*

REFLECTIONS

JOY TO EMBRACE	STRESS TO RELEASE	FOCUSING ON	GRATITUDE FOR

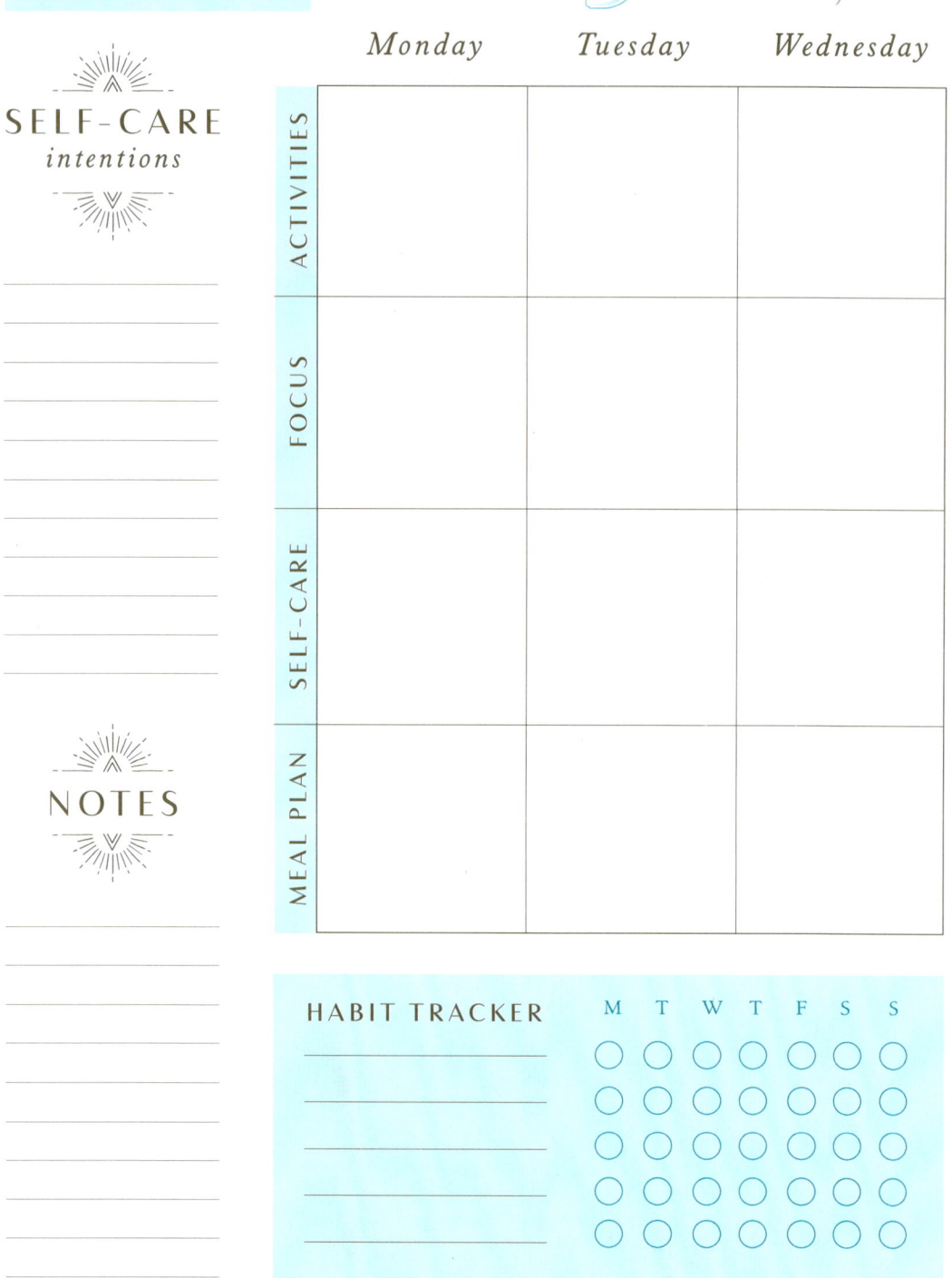

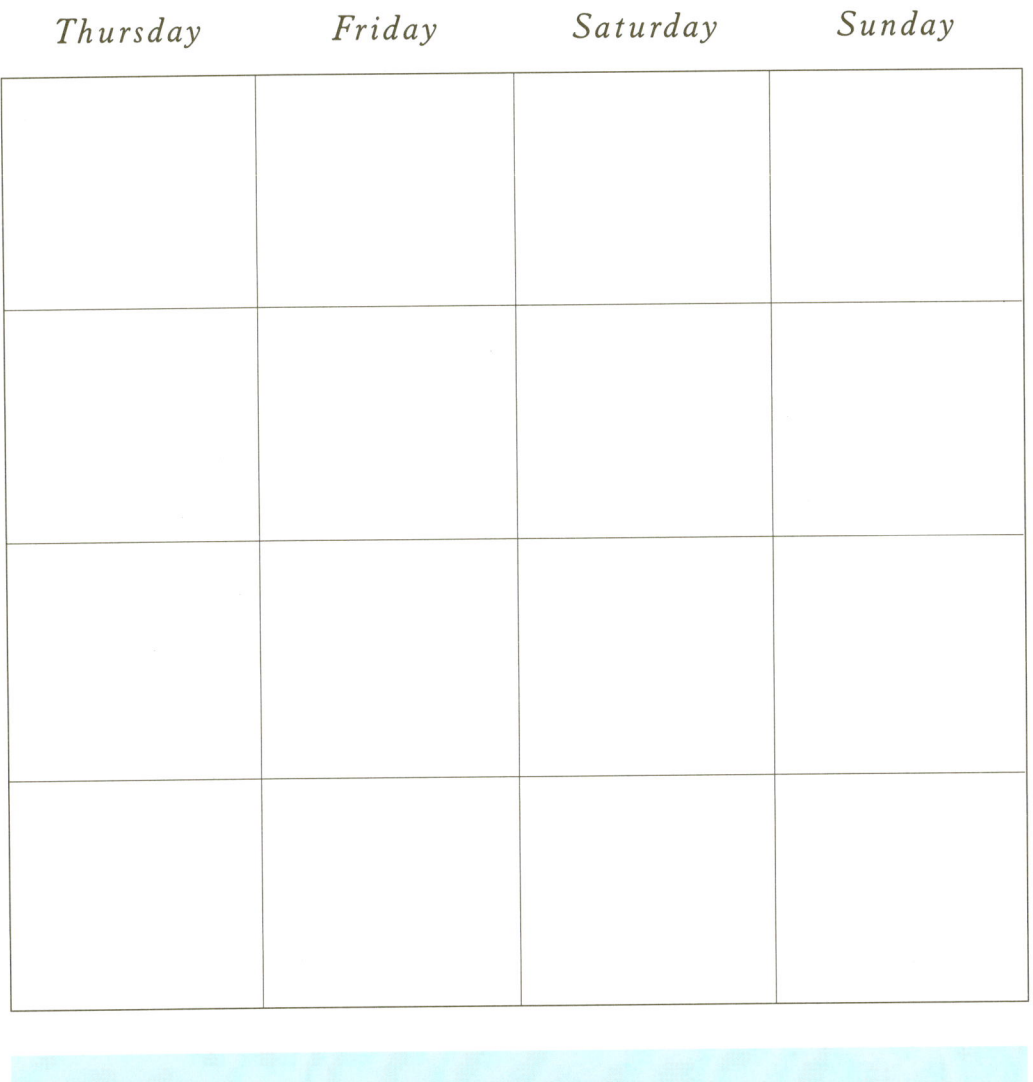

Thursday	Friday	Saturday	Sunday

REFLECTIONS

JOY TO EMBRACE	STRESS TO RELEASE	FOCUSING ON	GRATITUDE FOR

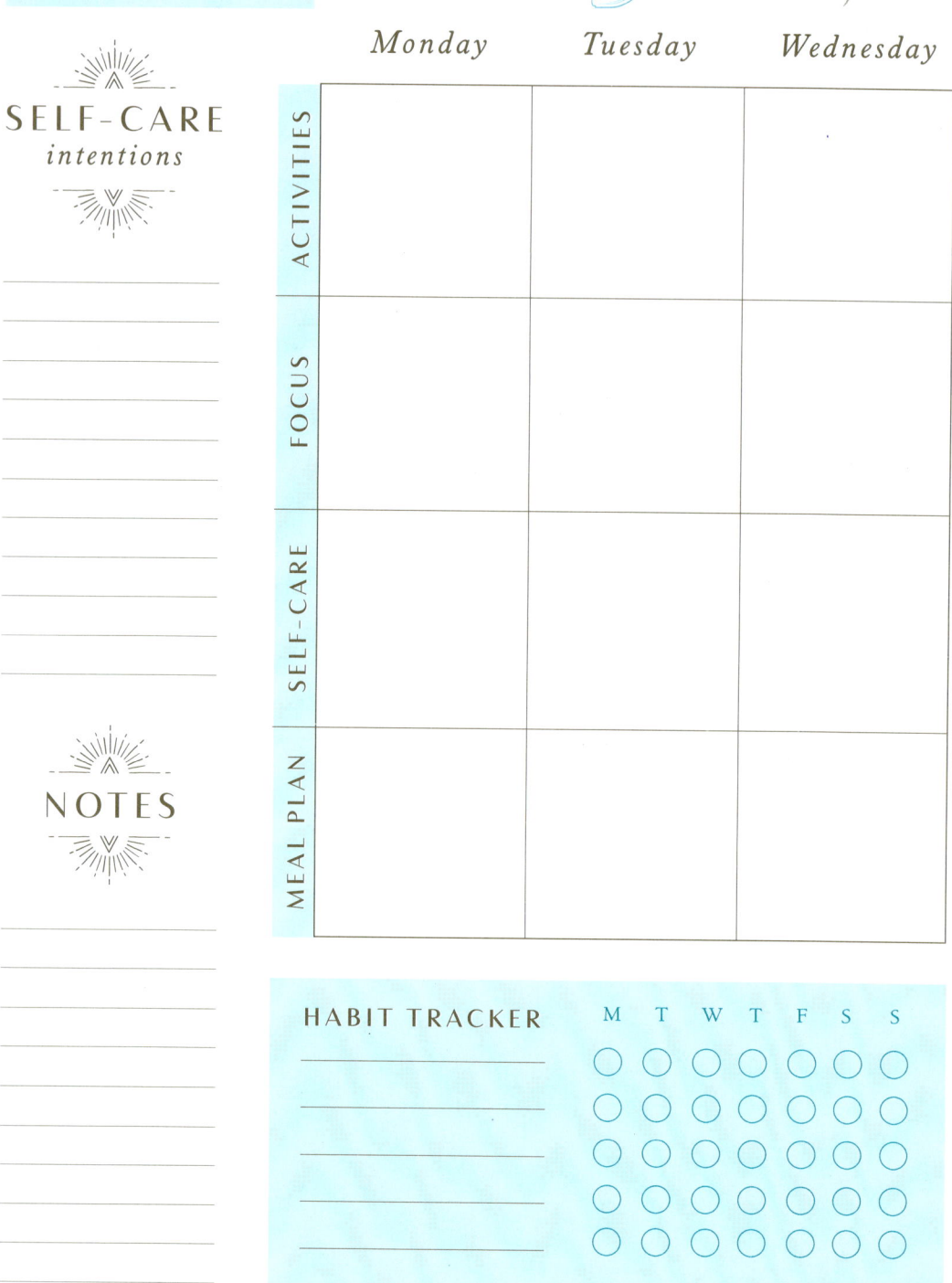

Thursday	*Friday*	*Saturday*	*Sunday*

REFLECTIONS

JOY TO EMBRACE	STRESS TO RELEASE	FOCUSING ON	GRATITUDE FOR

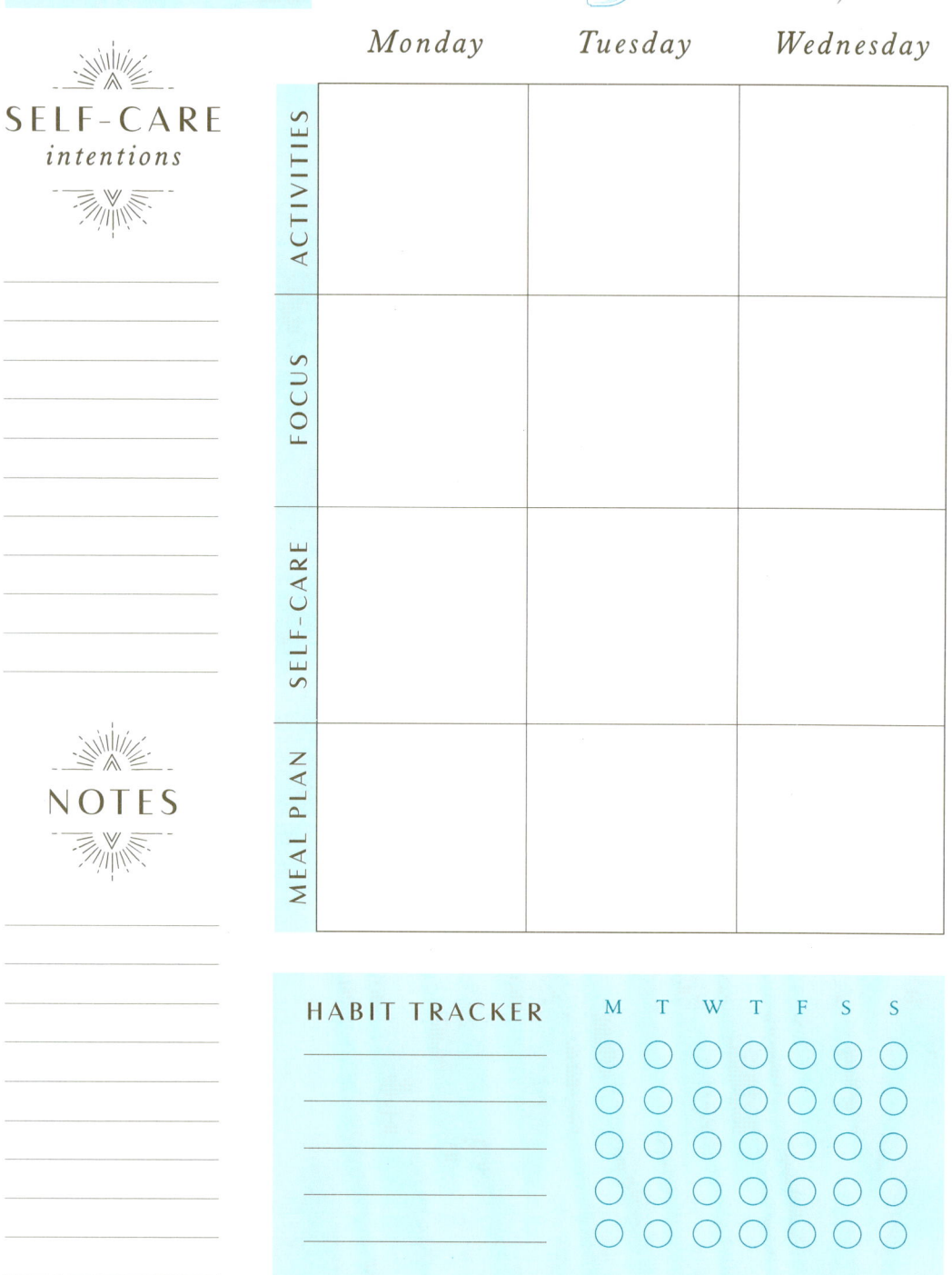

Thursday	Friday	Saturday	Sunday

REFLECTIONS

JOY TO EMBRACE	STRESS TO RELEASE	FOCUSING ON	GRATITUDE FOR

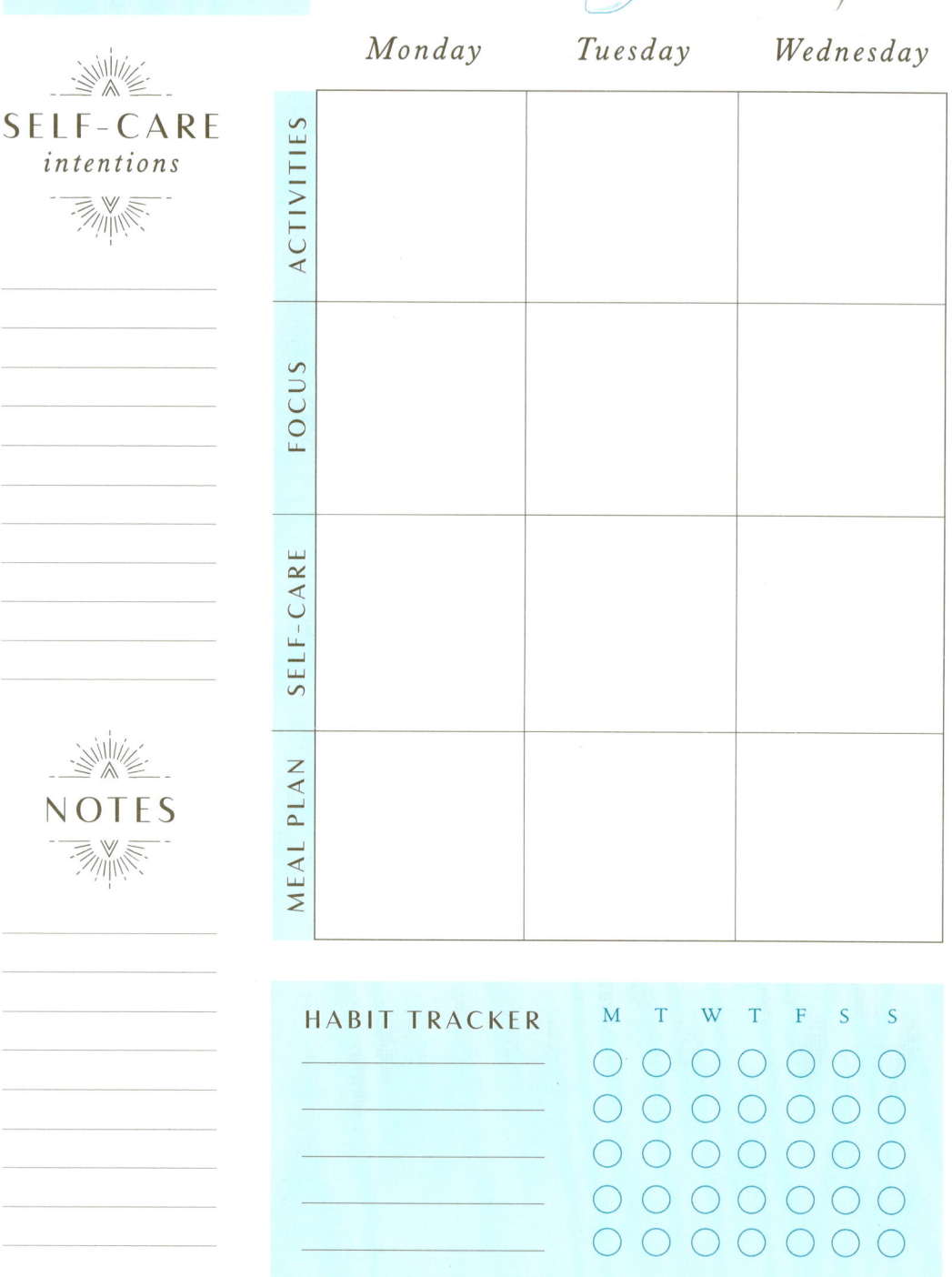

SELF-CARE
intentions

NOTES

	Monday	Tuesday	Wednesday
ACTIVITIES			
FOCUS			
SELF-CARE			
MEAL PLAN			

HABIT TRACKER

M T W T F S S

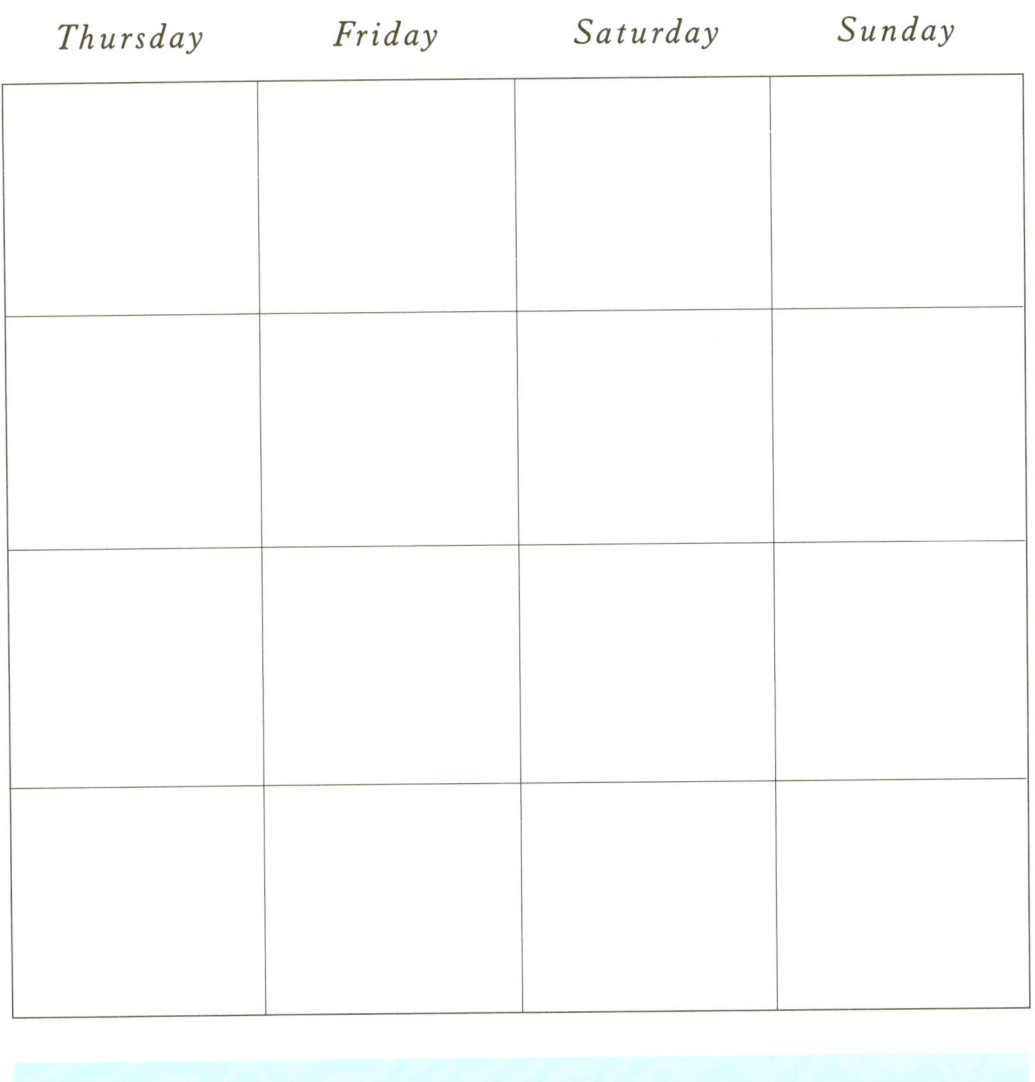

Thursday	Friday	Saturday	Sunday

REFLECTIONS

JOY TO EMBRACE	STRESS TO RELEASE	FOCUSING ON	GRATITUDE FOR

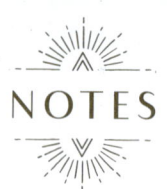

NOTES

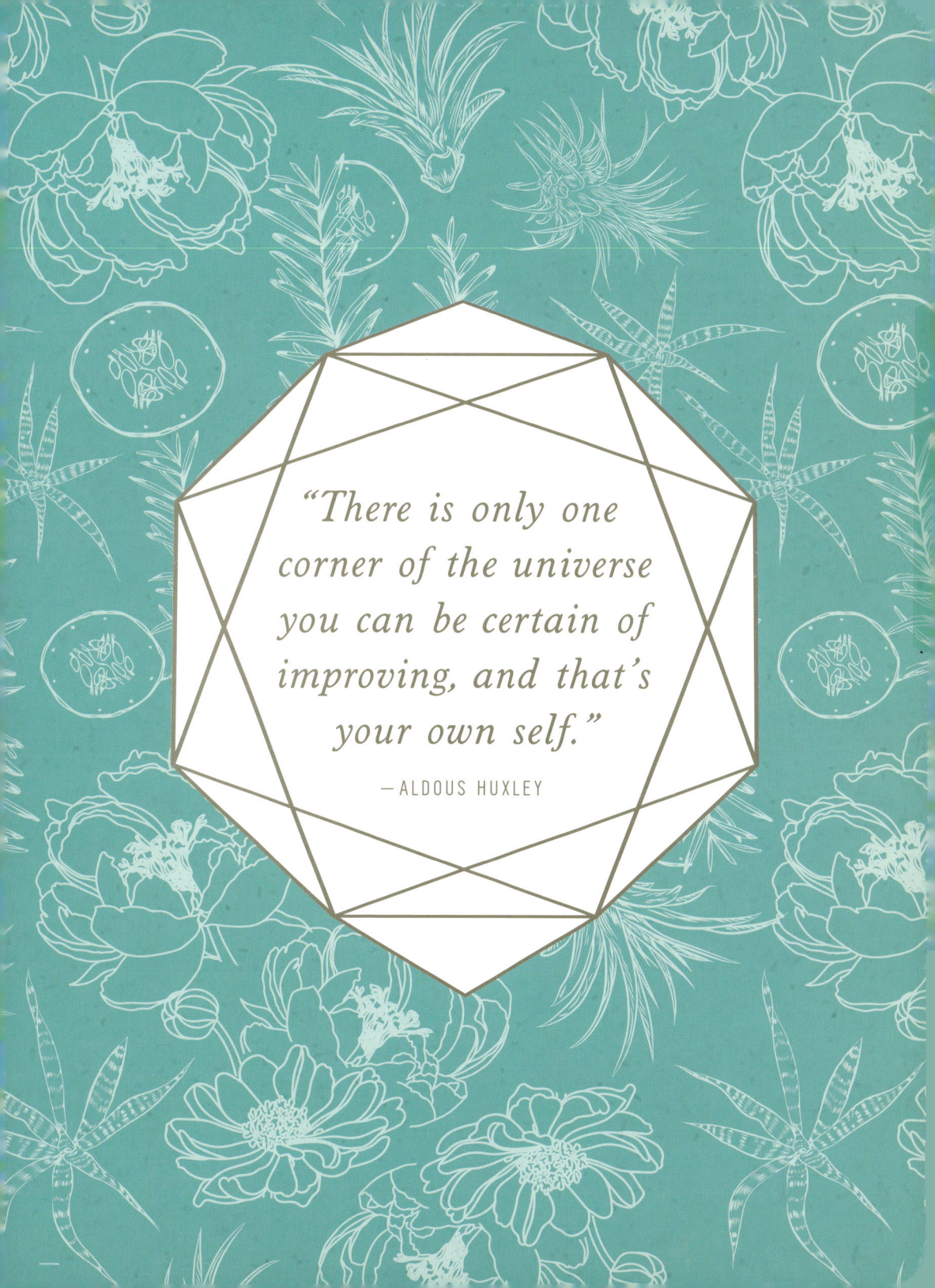

SELF-CARE
priorities

Monday | *Tuesday* | *Wednesday*

IT'S GOOD TO DO UNCOMFORTABLE THINGS. IT'S WEIGHT TRAINING FOR LIFE.
–Anne Lamott

NOTES

Thursday	Friday	Saturday	Sunday

BIRTHDAYS

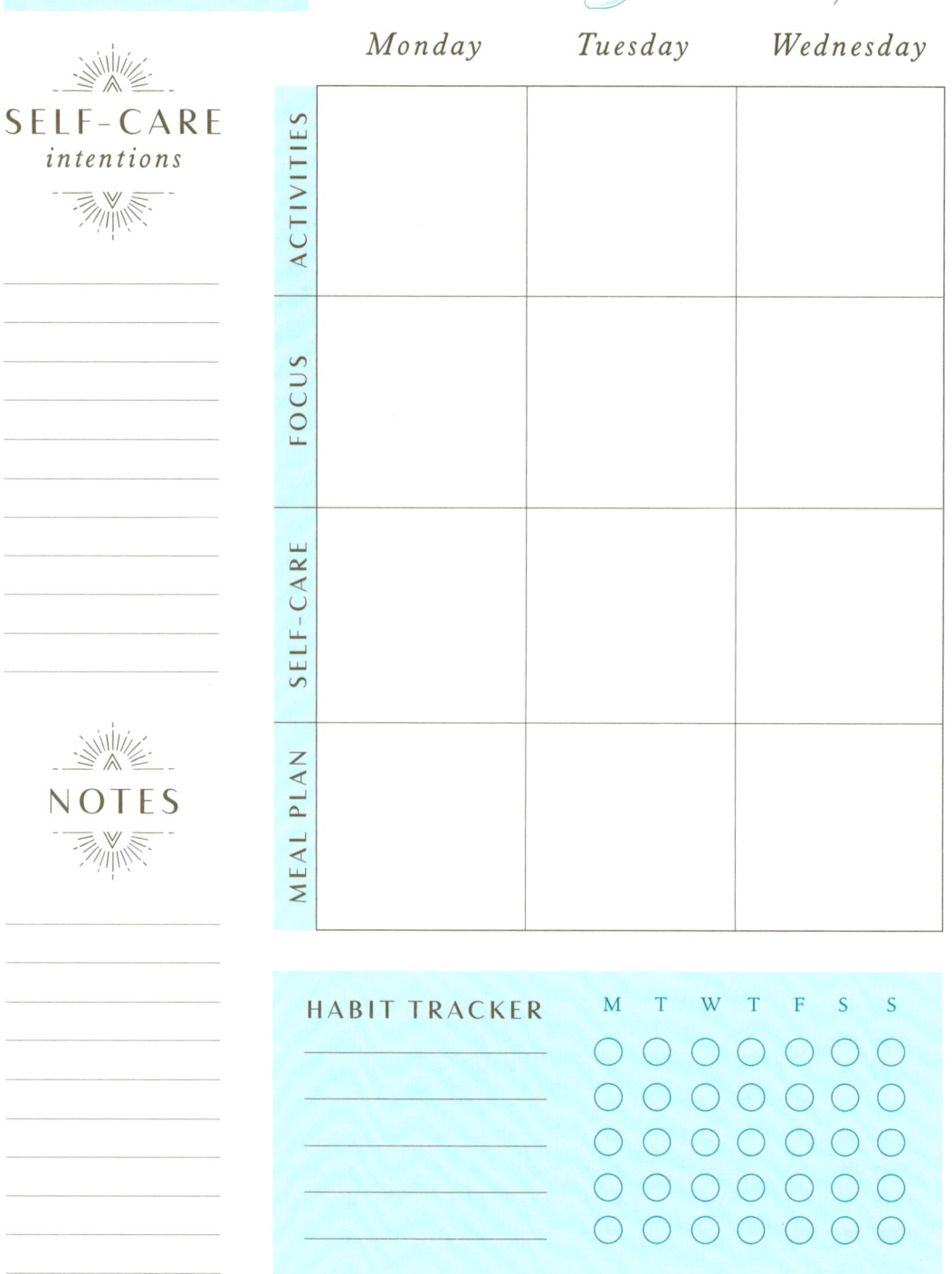

Thursday	Friday	Saturday	Sunday

REFLECTIONS

JOY TO EMBRACE	STRESS TO RELEASE	FOCUSING ON	GRATITUDE FOR

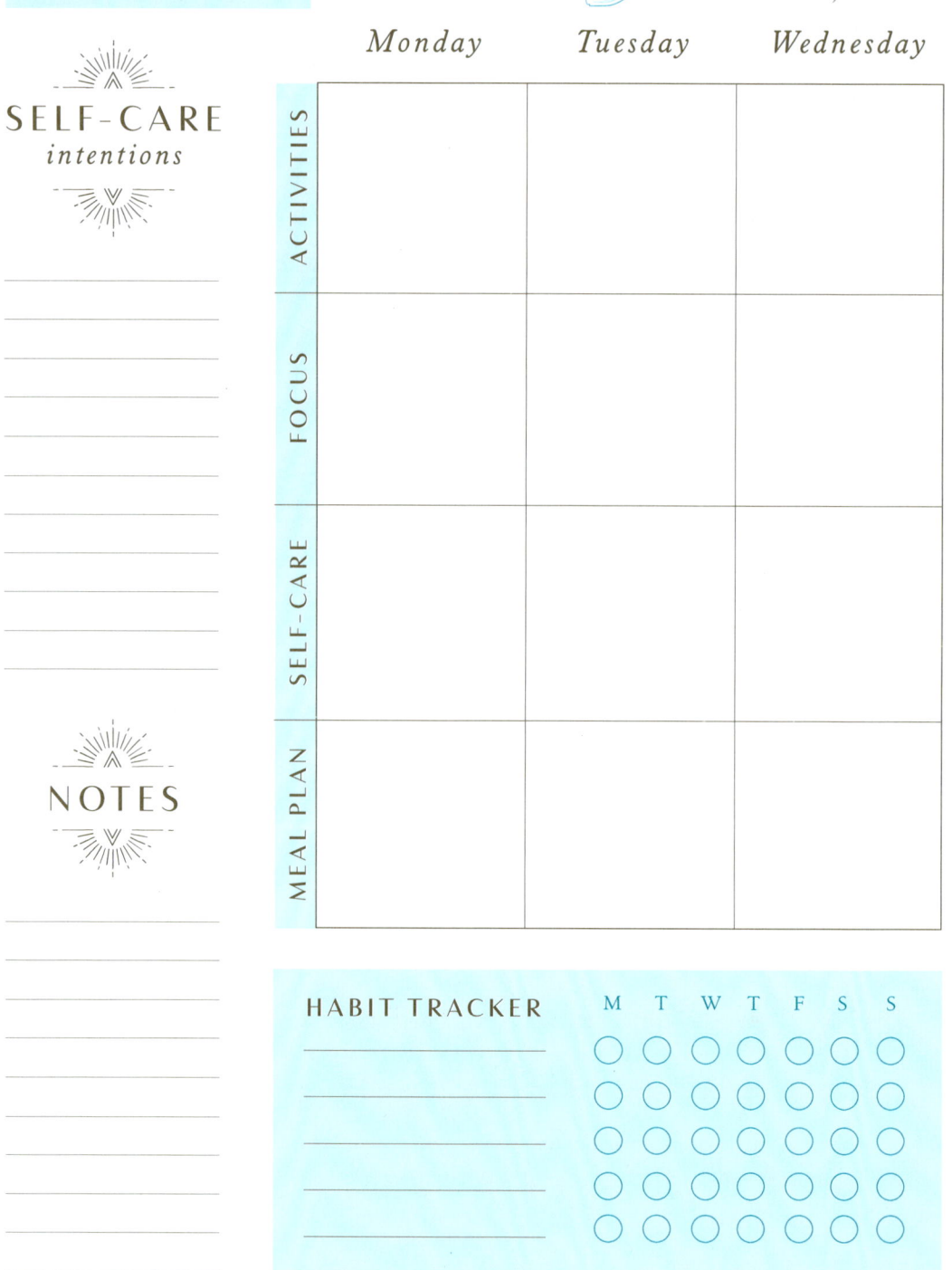

Thursday	Friday	Saturday	Sunday

REFLECTIONS

JOY TO EMBRACE	STRESS TO RELEASE	FOCUSING ON	GRATITUDE FOR

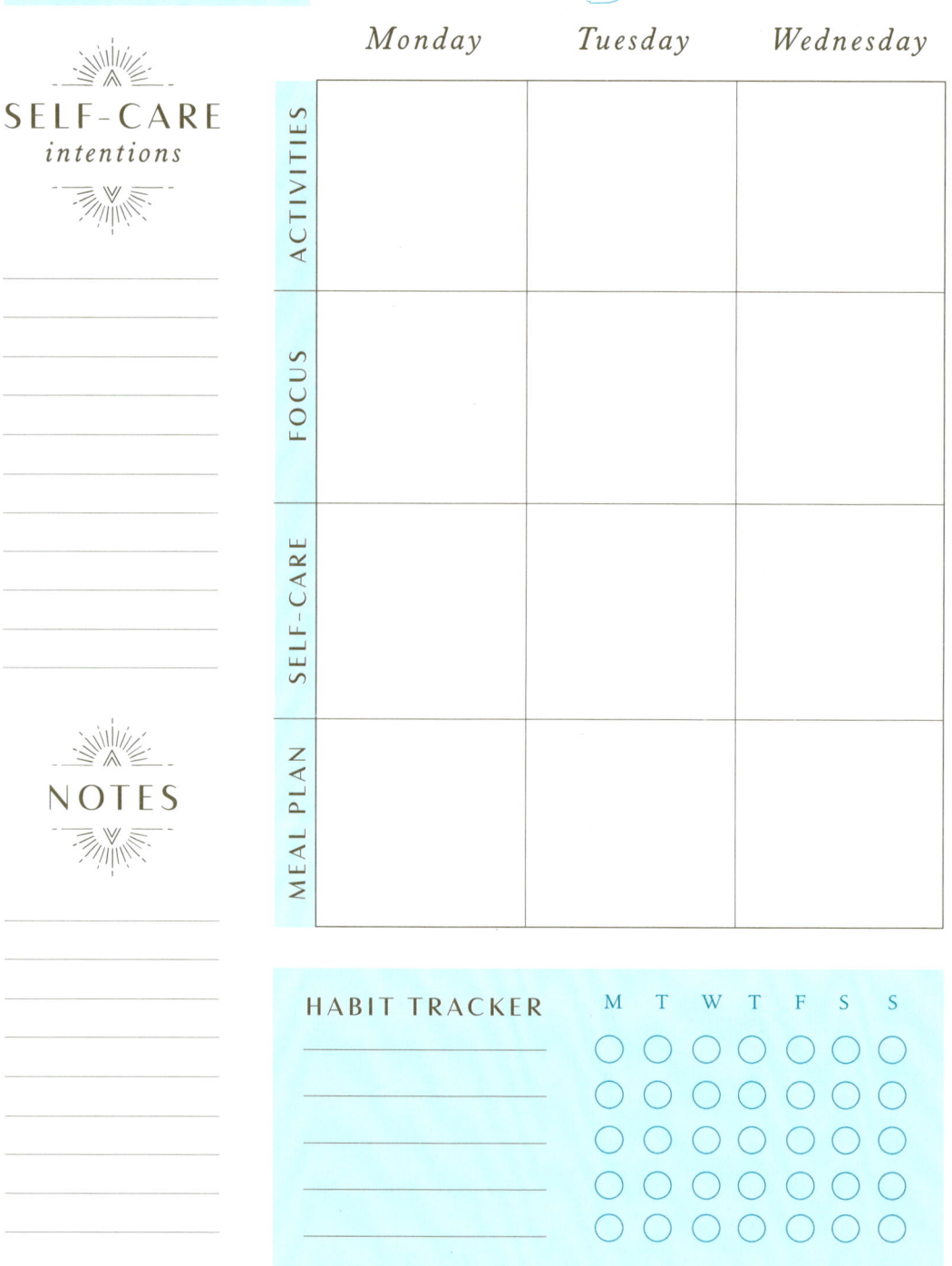

Thursday	*Friday*	*Saturday*	*Sunday*

REFLECTIONS

JOY TO EMBRACE	STRESS TO RELEASE	FOCUSING ON	GRATITUDE FOR

SELF-CARE
intentions

	Monday	Tuesday	Wednesday
ACTIVITIES			
FOCUS			
SELF-CARE			
MEAL PLAN			

NOTES

HABIT TRACKER

M T W T F S S
○ ○ ○ ○ ○ ○ ○
○ ○ ○ ○ ○ ○ ○
○ ○ ○ ○ ○ ○ ○
○ ○ ○ ○ ○ ○ ○
○ ○ ○ ○ ○ ○ ○

Thursday	Friday	Saturday	Sunday

REFLECTIONS

JOY TO EMBRACE	STRESS TO RELEASE	FOCUSING ON	GRATITUDE FOR

SELF-CARE
intentions

	Monday	Tuesday	Wednesday
ACTIVITIES			
FOCUS			
SELF-CARE			
MEAL PLAN			

NOTES

HABIT TRACKER

M T W T F S S

Thursday	Friday	Saturday	Sunday

REFLECTIONS

JOY TO EMBRACE	STRESS TO RELEASE	FOCUSING ON	GRATITUDE FOR

NOTES

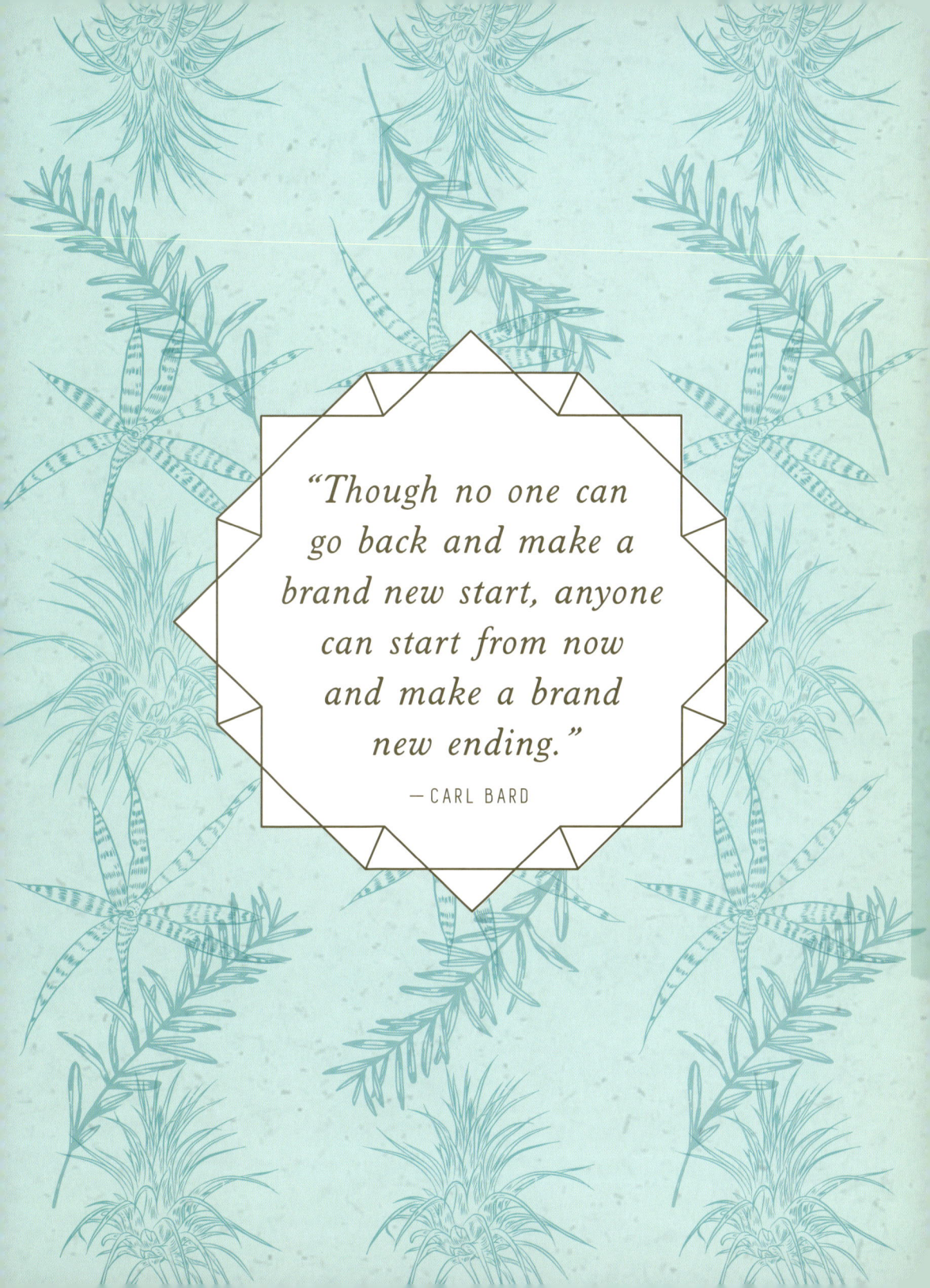

"Though no one can go back and make a brand new start, anyone can start from now and make a brand new ending."

— CARL BARD

SELF-CARE
priorities

_____
_____
_____
_____
_____
_____
_____
_____
_____
_____
_____
_____

TAKE CARE OF YOUR BODY. IT'S THE ONLY PLACE YOU HAVE TO LIVE.
–Jim Rohn

Monday	*Tuesday*	*Wednesday*

NOTES

Thursday	Friday	Saturday	Sunday

BIRTHDAYS

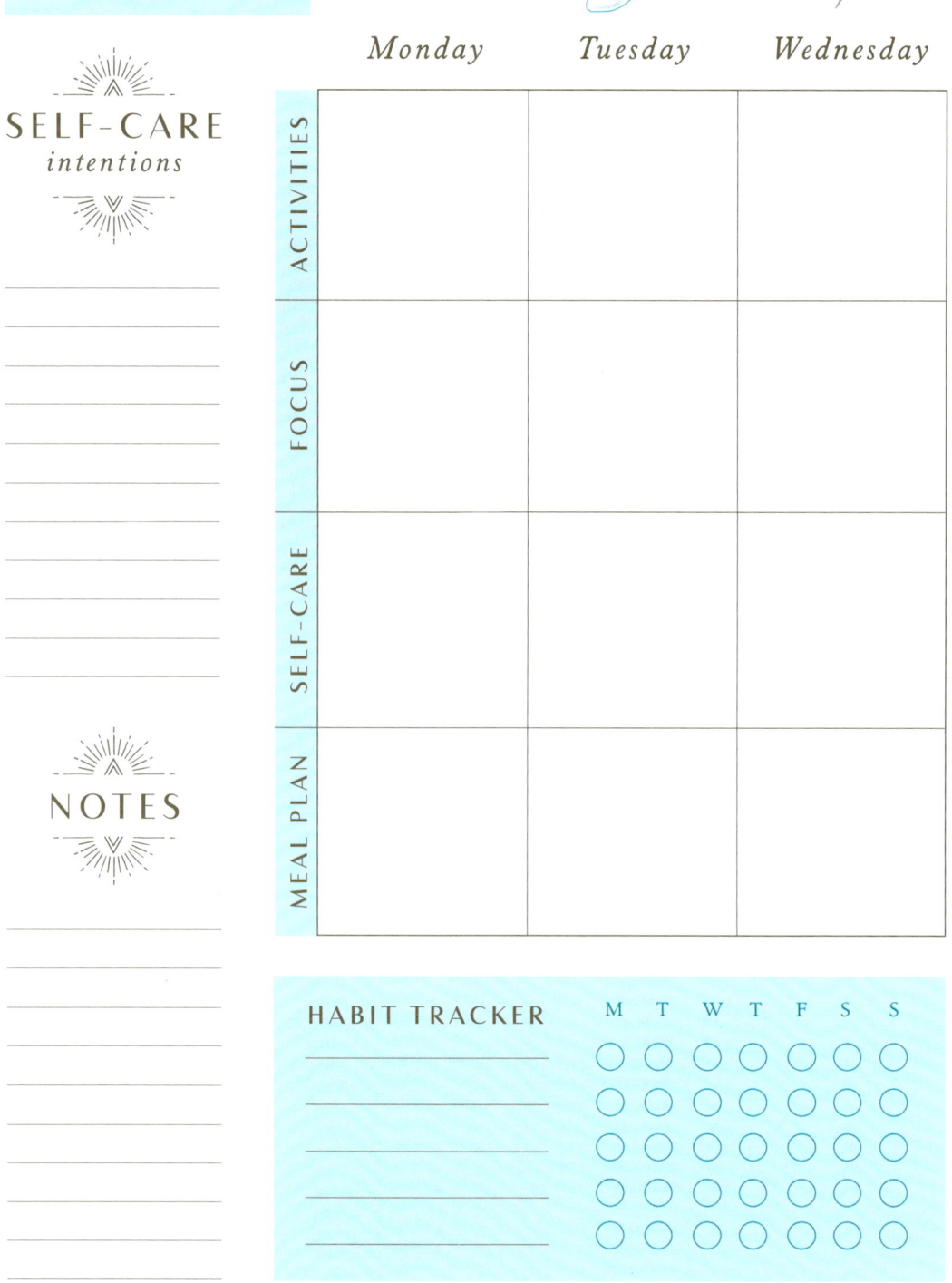

Thursday	*Friday*	*Saturday*	*Sunday*

REFLECTIONS

JOY TO EMBRACE	STRESS TO RELEASE	FOCUSING ON	GRATITUDE FOR

SELF-CARE
intentions

	Monday	Tuesday	Wednesday
ACTIVITIES			
FOCUS			
SELF-CARE			
MEAL PLAN			

NOTES

HABIT TRACKER

	M	T	W	T	F	S	S
	○	○	○	○	○	○	○
	○	○	○	○	○	○	○
	○	○	○	○	○	○	○
	○	○	○	○	○	○	○
	○	○	○	○	○	○	○

Thursday	Friday	Saturday	Sunday

REFLECTIONS

JOY TO EMBRACE	STRESS TO RELEASE	FOCUSING ON	GRATITUDE FOR

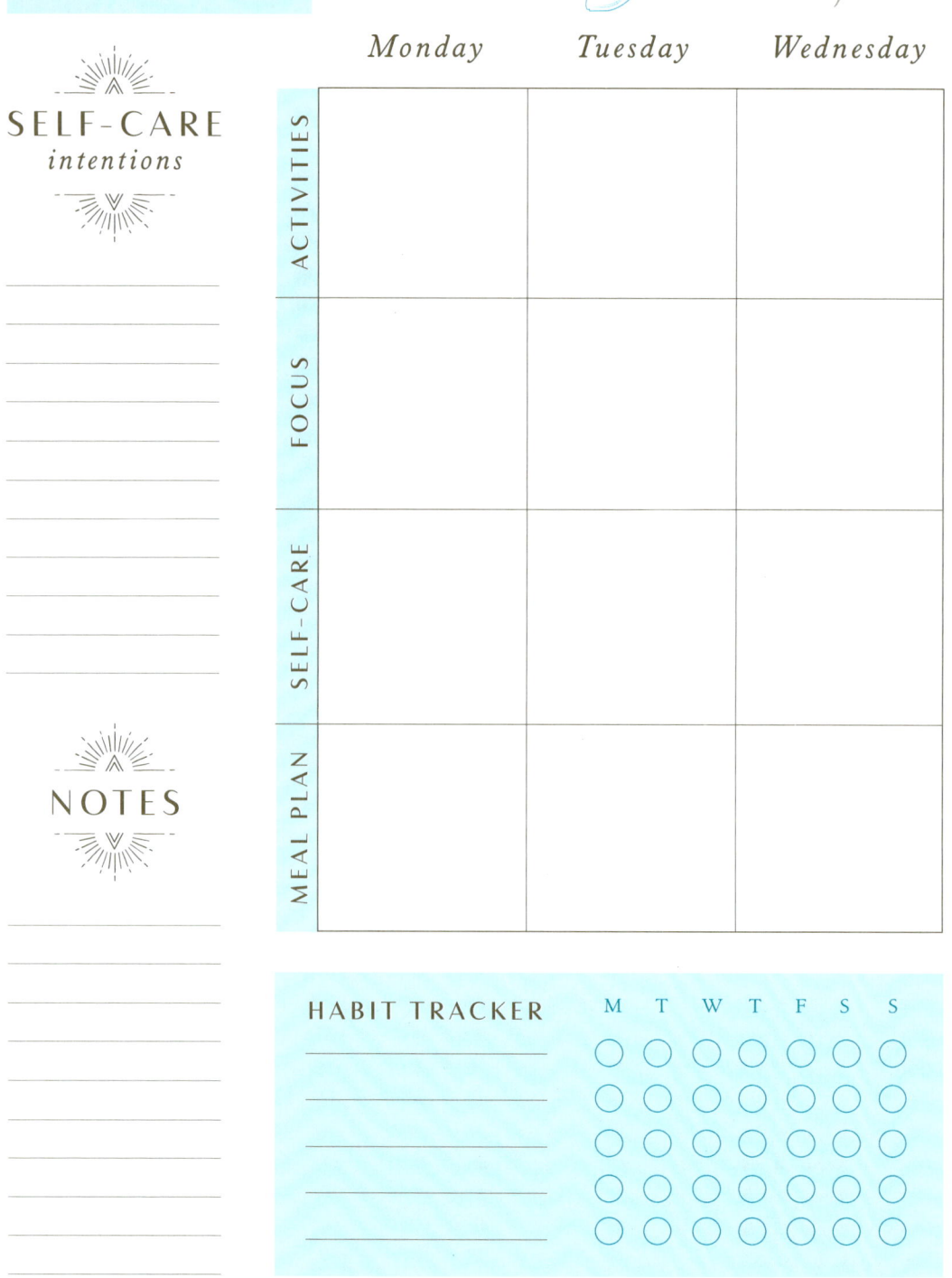

Thursday	Friday	Saturday	Sunday

REFLECTIONS

JOY TO EMBRACE	STRESS TO RELEASE	FOCUSING ON	GRATITUDE FOR

SELF-CARE
intentions

	Monday	Tuesday	Wednesday
ACTIVITIES			
FOCUS			
SELF-CARE			
MEAL PLAN			

NOTES

HABIT TRACKER

	M	T	W	T	F	S	S
	○	○	○	○	○	○	○
	○	○	○	○	○	○	○
	○	○	○	○	○	○	○
	○	○	○	○	○	○	○
	○	○	○	○	○	○	○

Thursday	Friday	Saturday	Sunday

REFLECTIONS

JOY TO EMBRACE	STRESS TO RELEASE	FOCUSING ON	GRATITUDE FOR

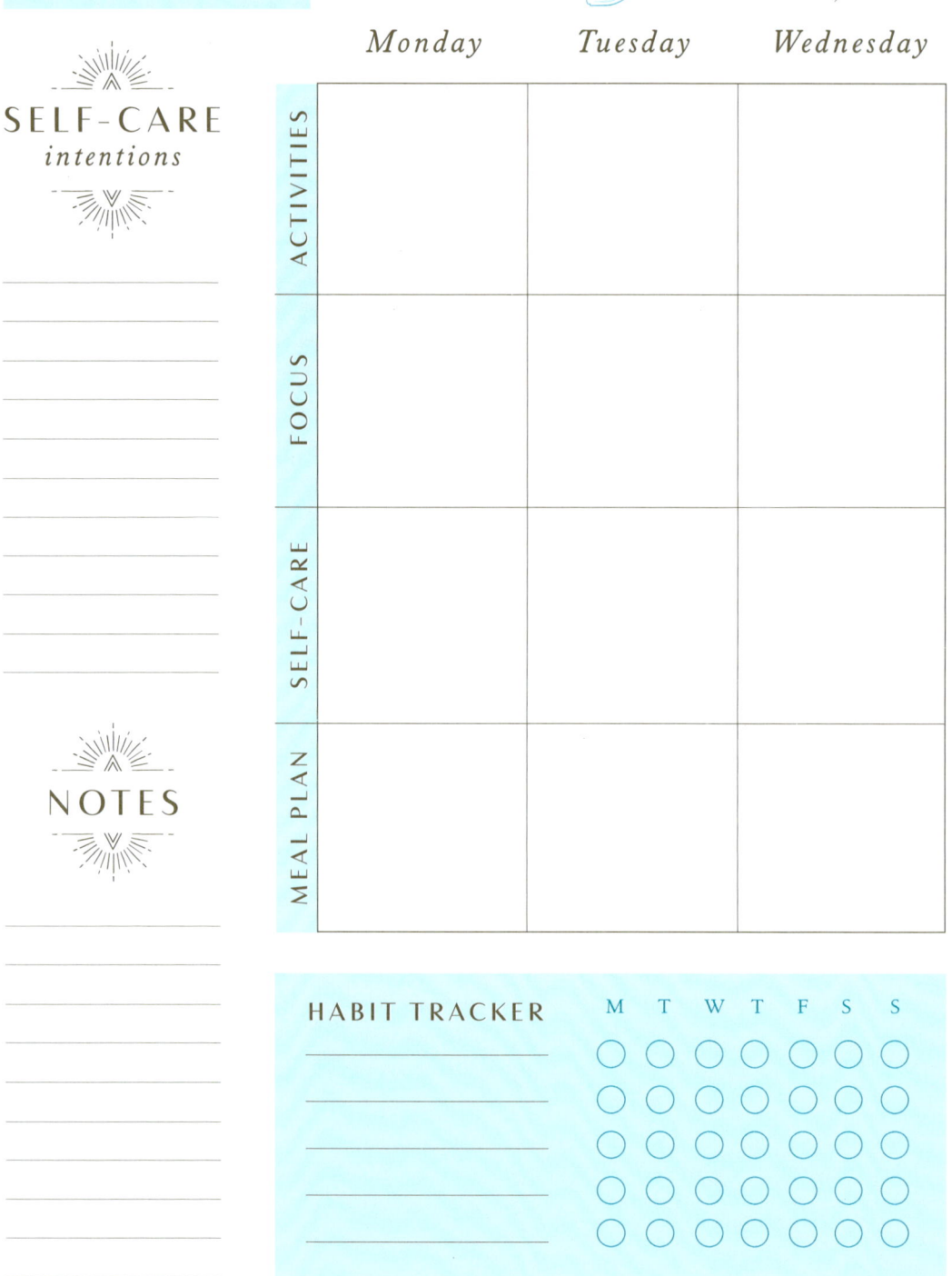

Thursday	Friday	Saturday	Sunday

REFLECTIONS

JOY TO EMBRACE	STRESS TO RELEASE	FOCUSING ON	GRATITUDE FOR

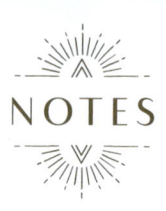

NOTES

> "Carve out and claim time to care for yourself and kindle your own fire."
>
> — AMY IPPOLITI

SELF-CARE
priorities

	Monday	Tuesday	Wednesday

TAKE TIME OFF . . . THE WORLD WILL NOT FALL APART WITHOUT YOU.
—*Malebo Sephodi*

NOTES

Thursday	Friday	Saturday	Sunday

BIRTHDAYS

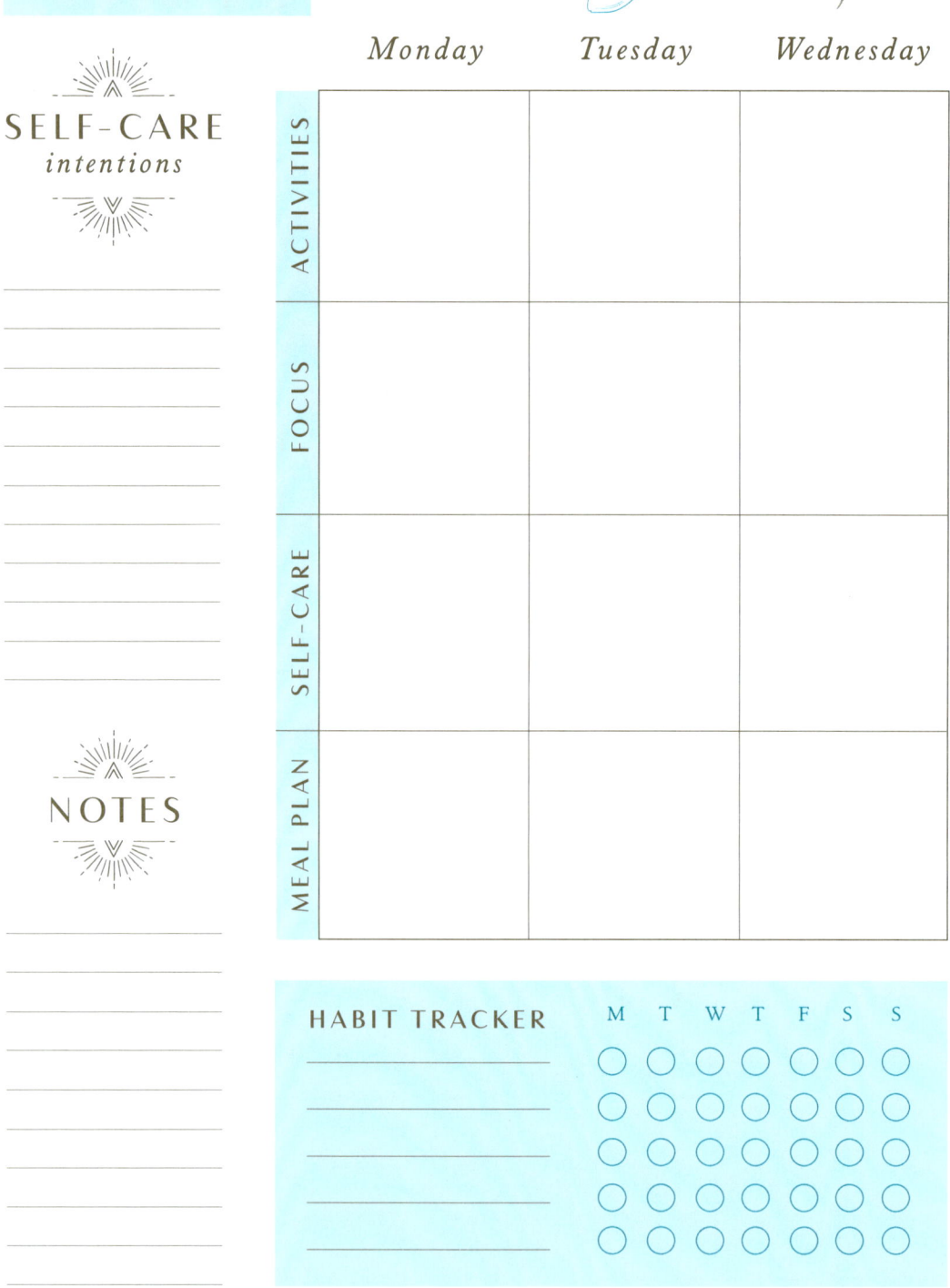

Thursday	*Friday*	*Saturday*	*Sunday*

REFLECTIONS

JOY TO EMBRACE	STRESS TO RELEASE	FOCUSING ON	GRATITUDE FOR

SELF-CARE
intentions

	Monday	Tuesday	Wednesday
ACTIVITIES			
FOCUS			
SELF-CARE			
MEAL PLAN			

NOTES

HABIT TRACKER

M T W T F S S
○ ○ ○ ○ ○ ○ ○
○ ○ ○ ○ ○ ○ ○
○ ○ ○ ○ ○ ○ ○
○ ○ ○ ○ ○ ○ ○
○ ○ ○ ○ ○ ○ ○

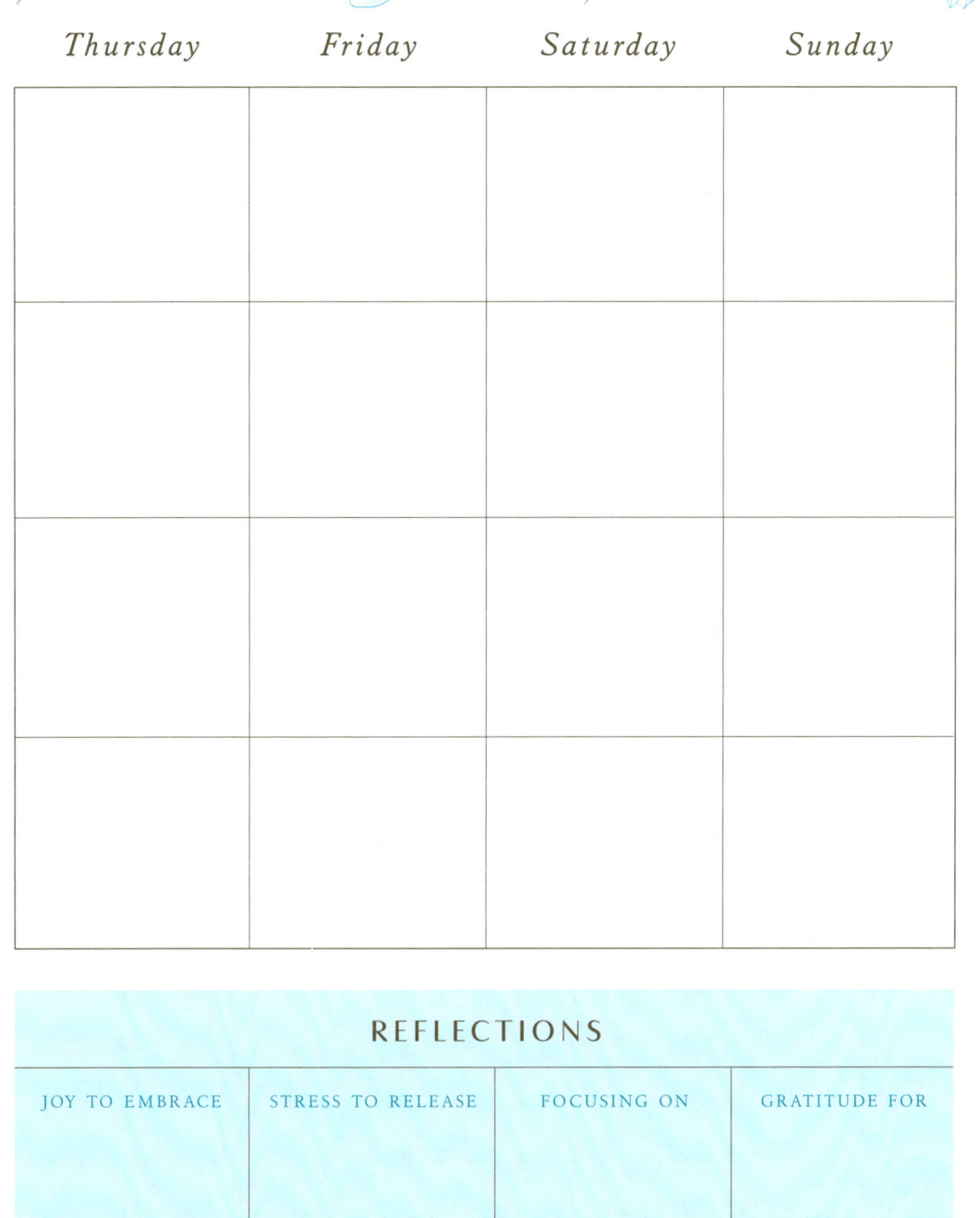

Thursday	Friday	Saturday	Sunday

REFLECTIONS

JOY TO EMBRACE	STRESS TO RELEASE	FOCUSING ON	GRATITUDE FOR

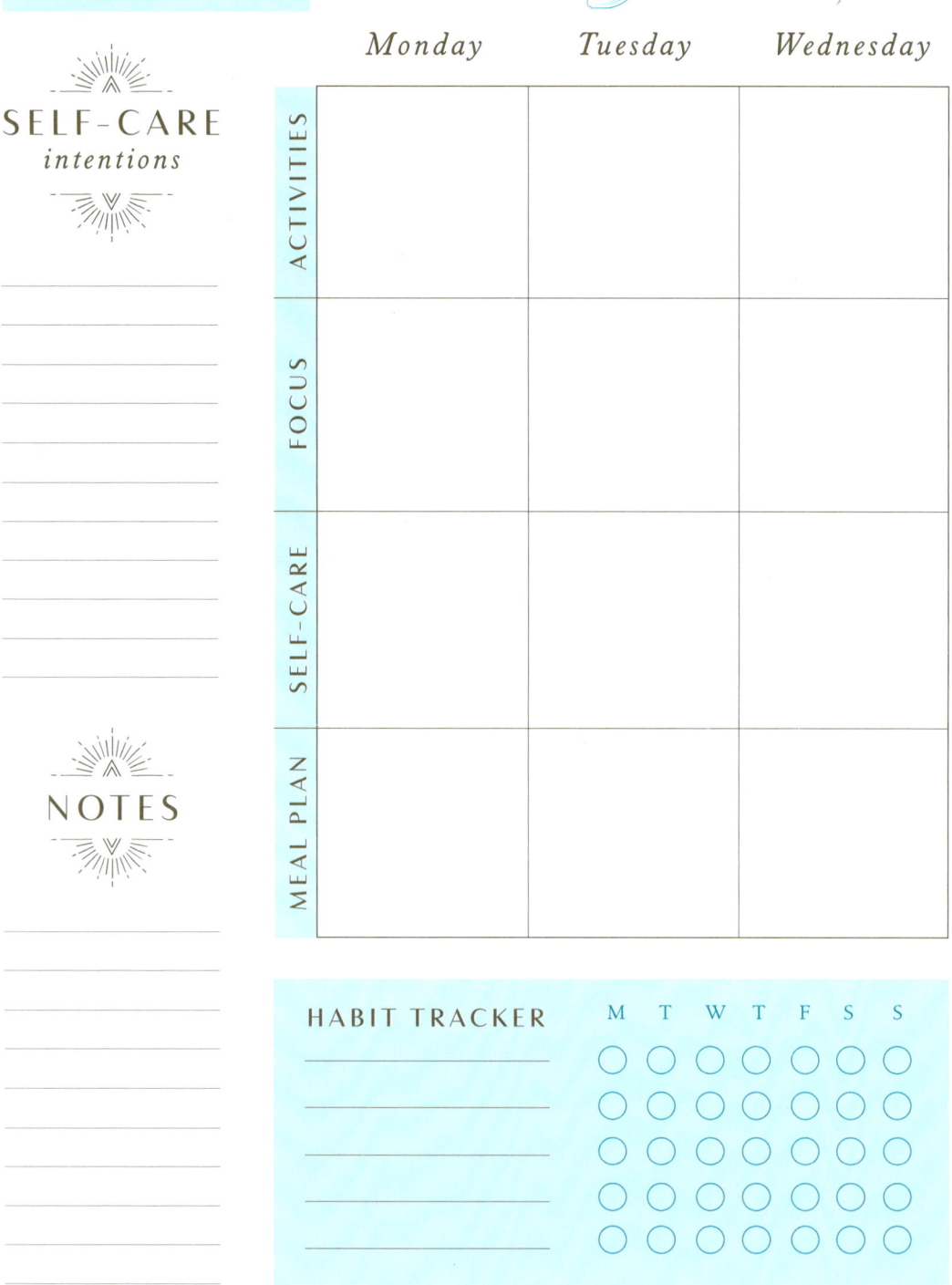

Thursday	Friday	Saturday	Sunday

REFLECTIONS

JOY TO EMBRACE	STRESS TO RELEASE	FOCUSING ON	GRATITUDE FOR

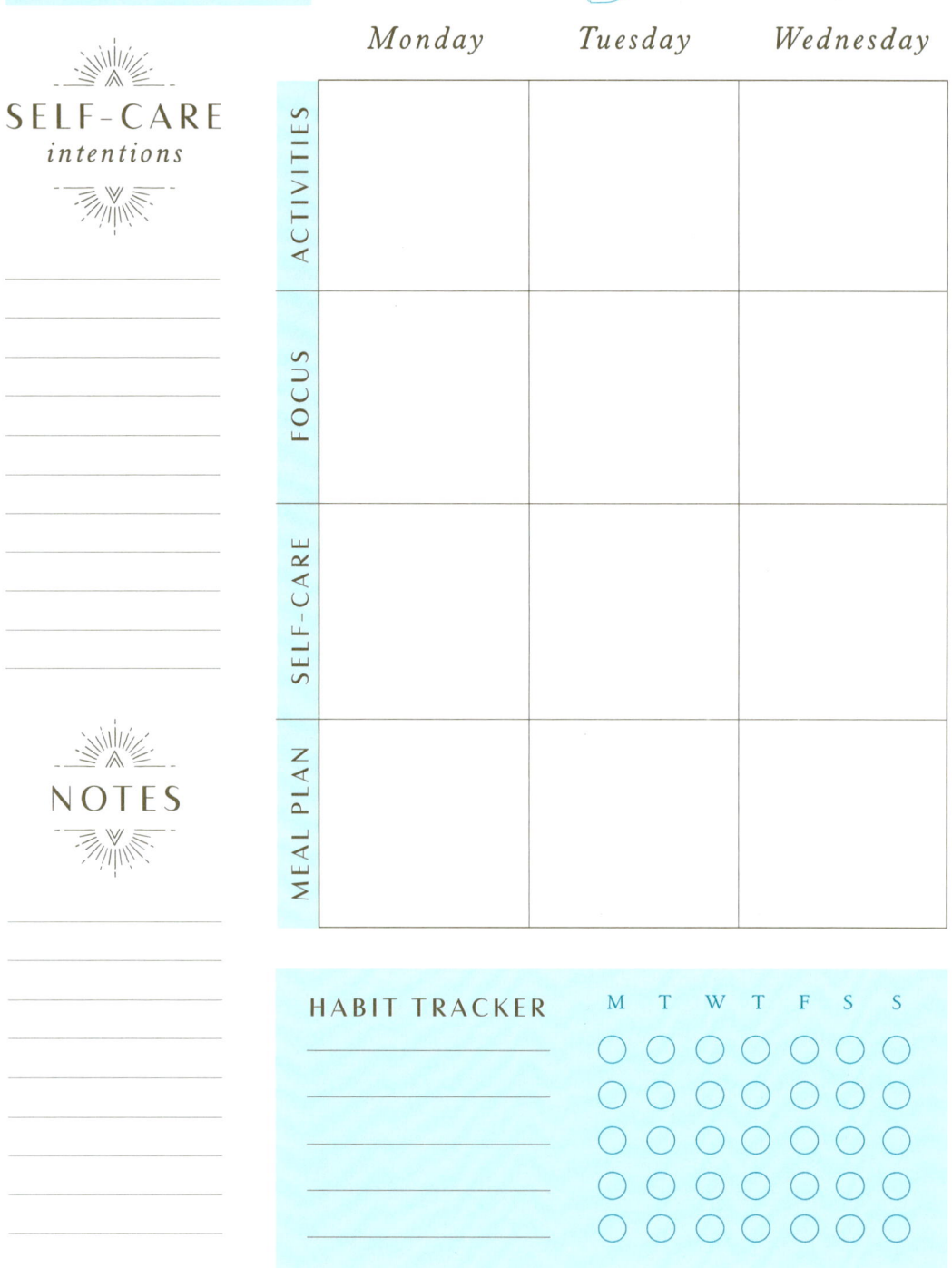

Thursday	Friday	Saturday	Sunday

REFLECTIONS

JOY TO EMBRACE	STRESS TO RELEASE	FOCUSING ON	GRATITUDE FOR

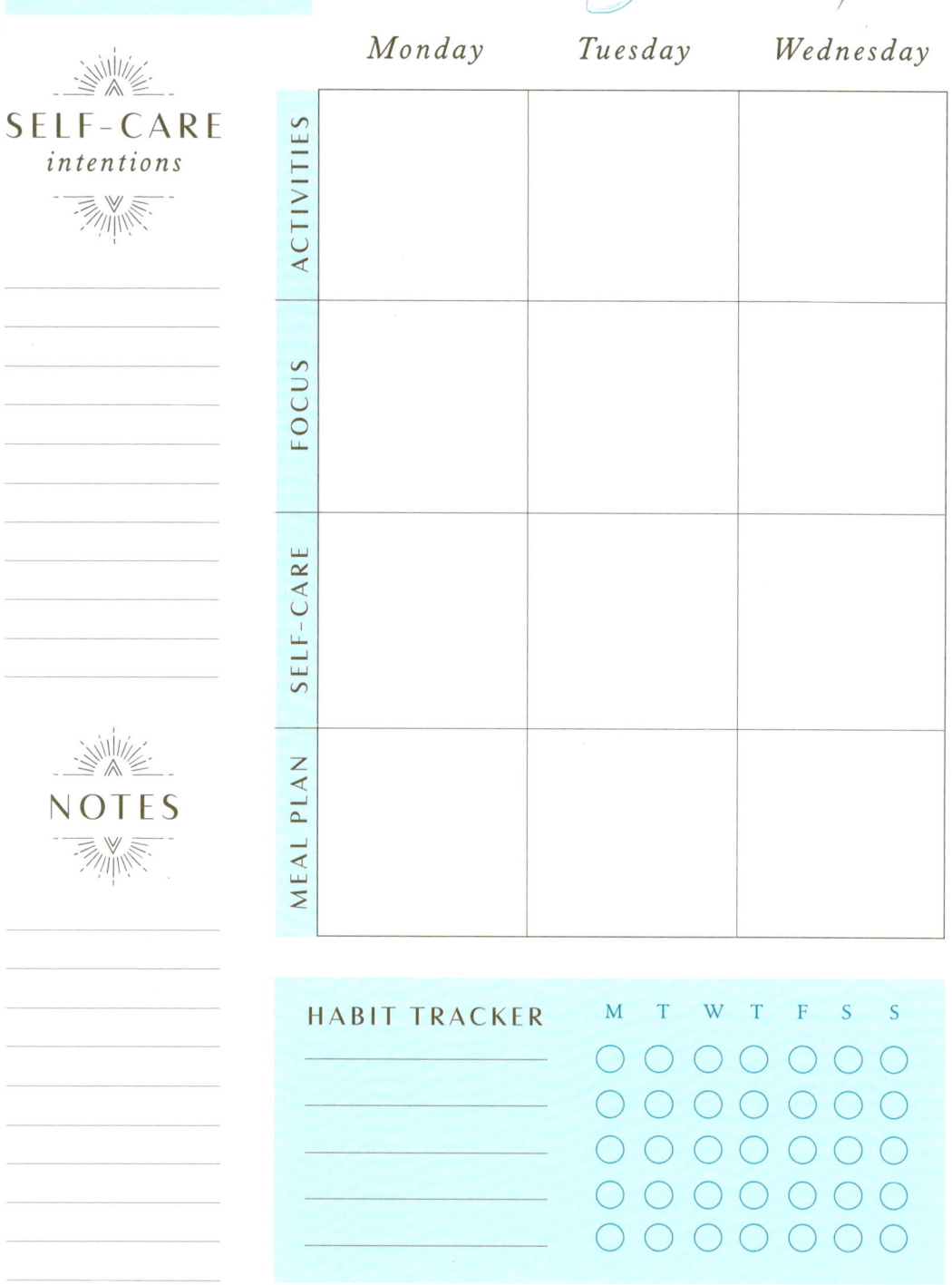

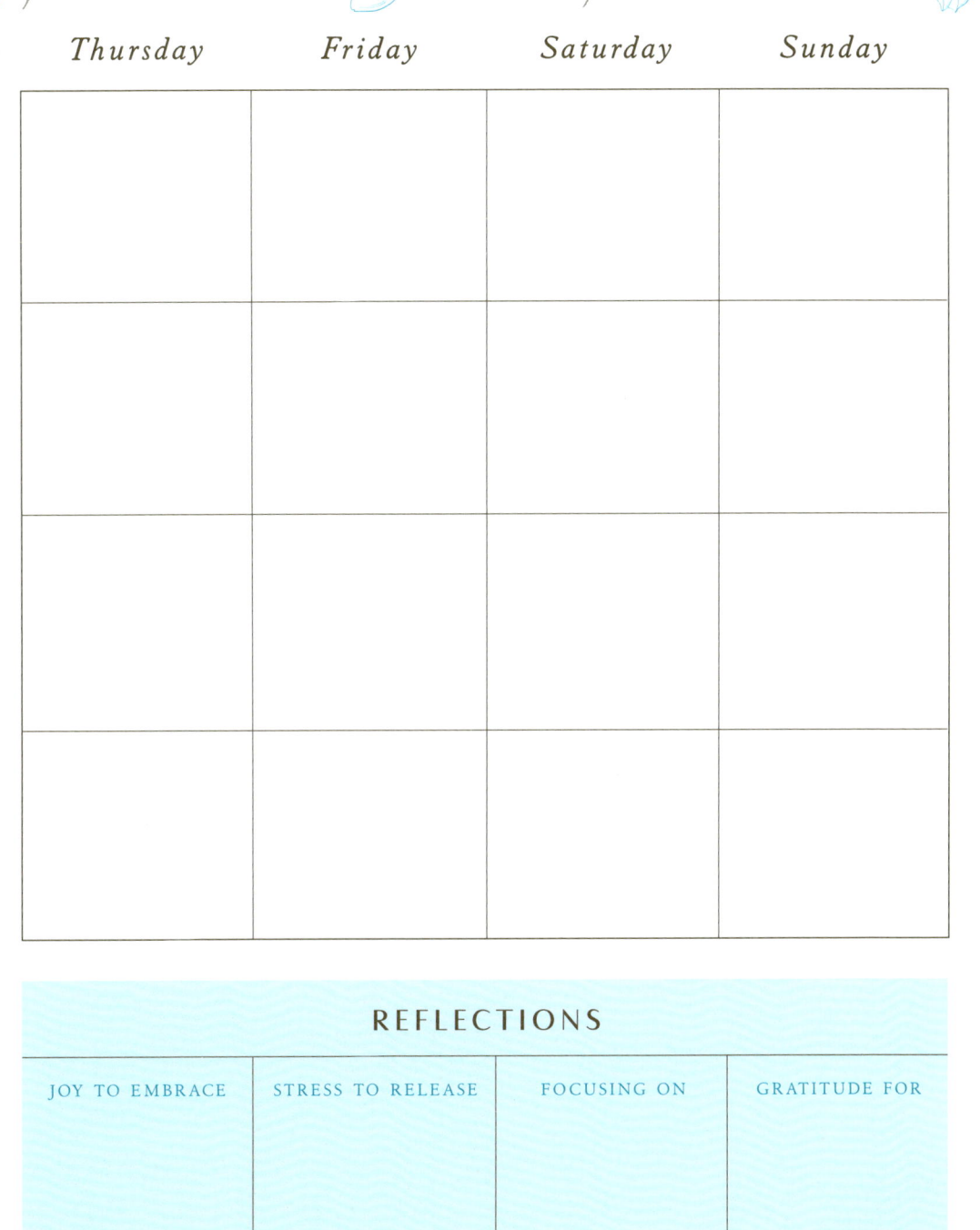

Thursday	Friday	Saturday	Sunday

REFLECTIONS

JOY TO EMBRACE	STRESS TO RELEASE	FOCUSING ON	GRATITUDE FOR

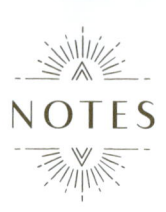

NOTES

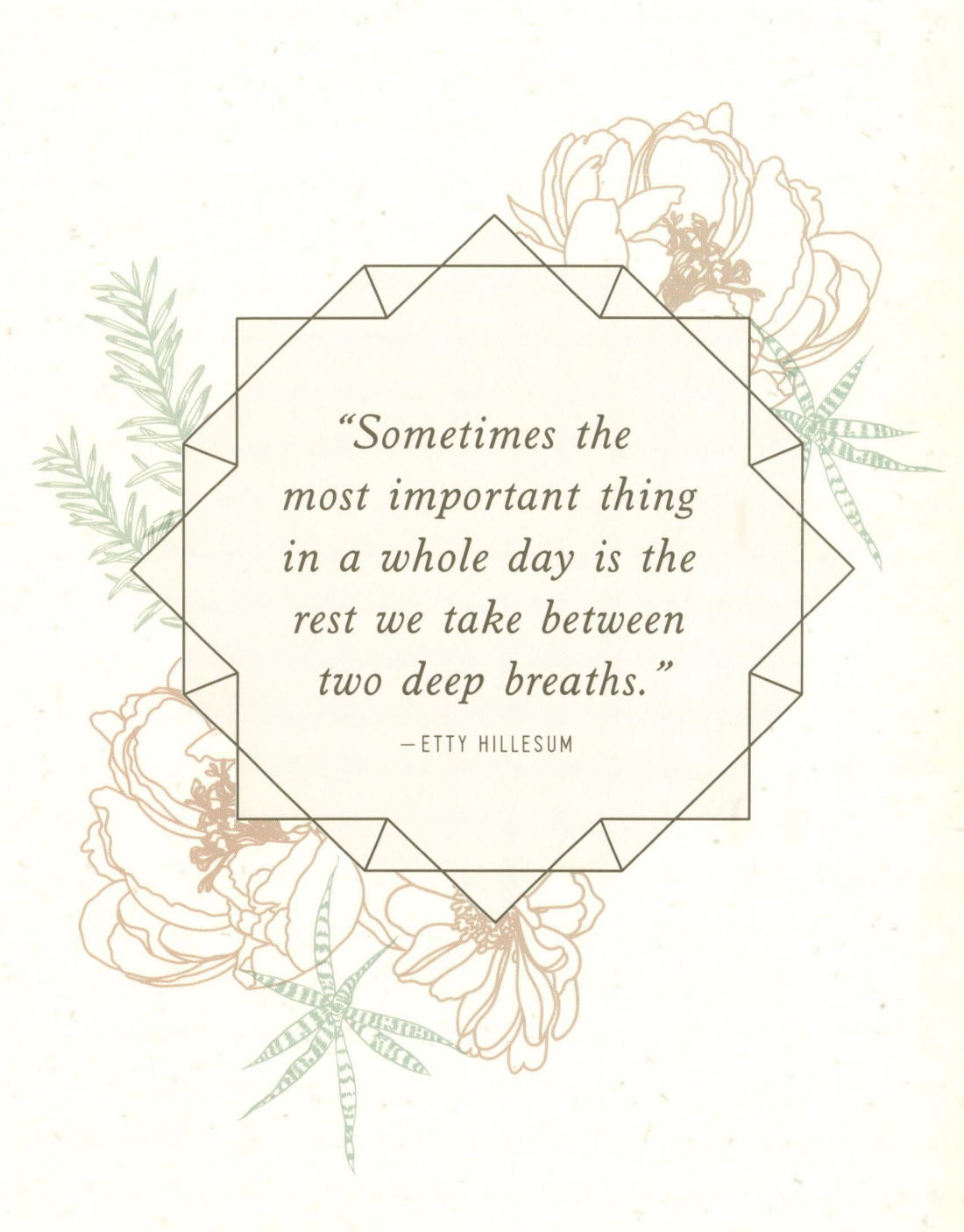

SELF-CARE
priorities

	Monday	Tuesday	Wednesday

TAKE CARE OF YOUR MIND, YOUR BODY WILL THANK YOU. TAKE CARE OF YOUR BODY, YOUR MIND WILL THANK YOU.
—*Debbie Hampton*

NOTES

Thursday	Friday	Saturday	Sunday

BIRTHDAYS

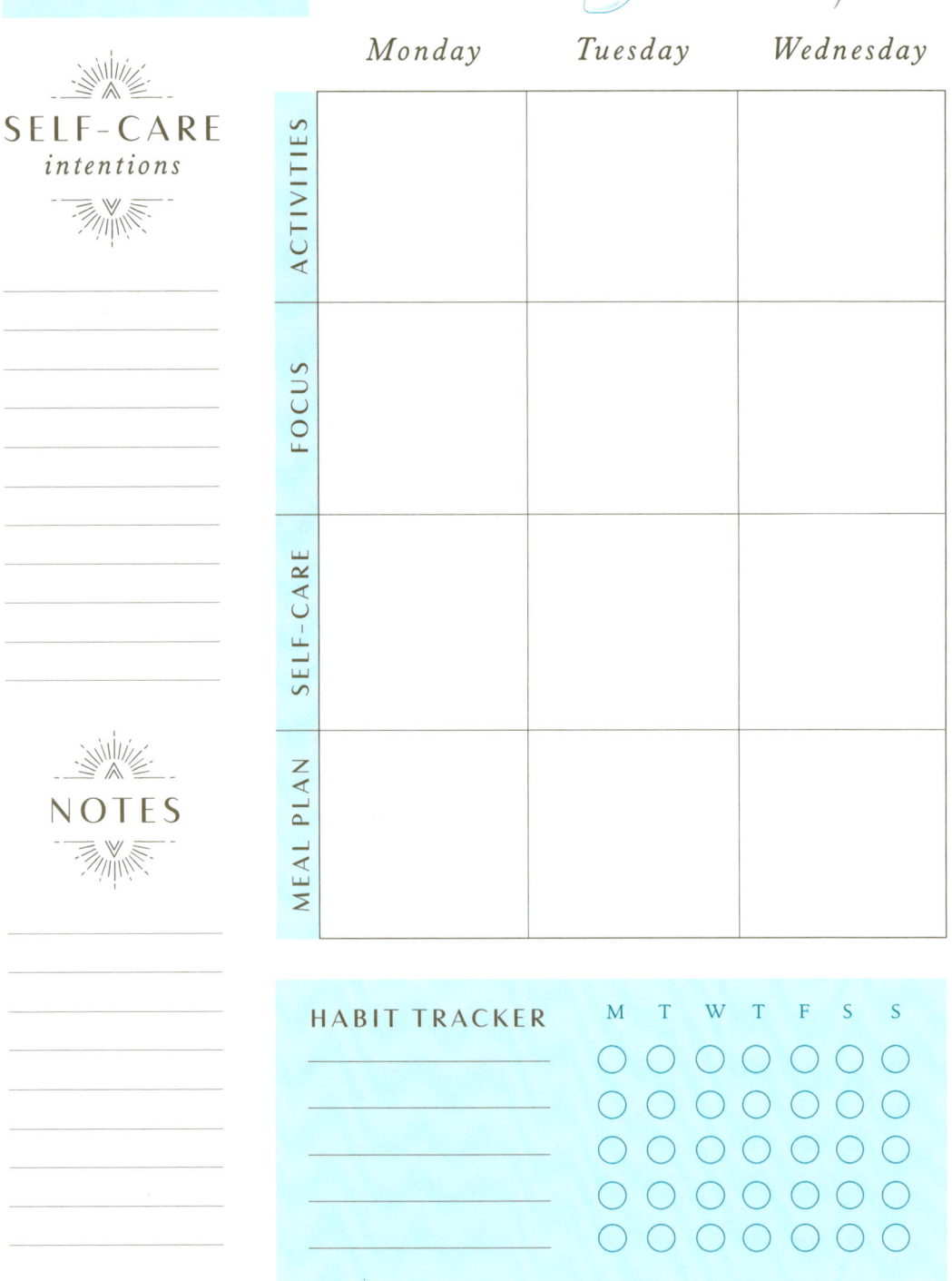

Thursday	Friday	Saturday	Sunday

REFLECTIONS

JOY TO EMBRACE	STRESS TO RELEASE	FOCUSING ON	GRATITUDE FOR

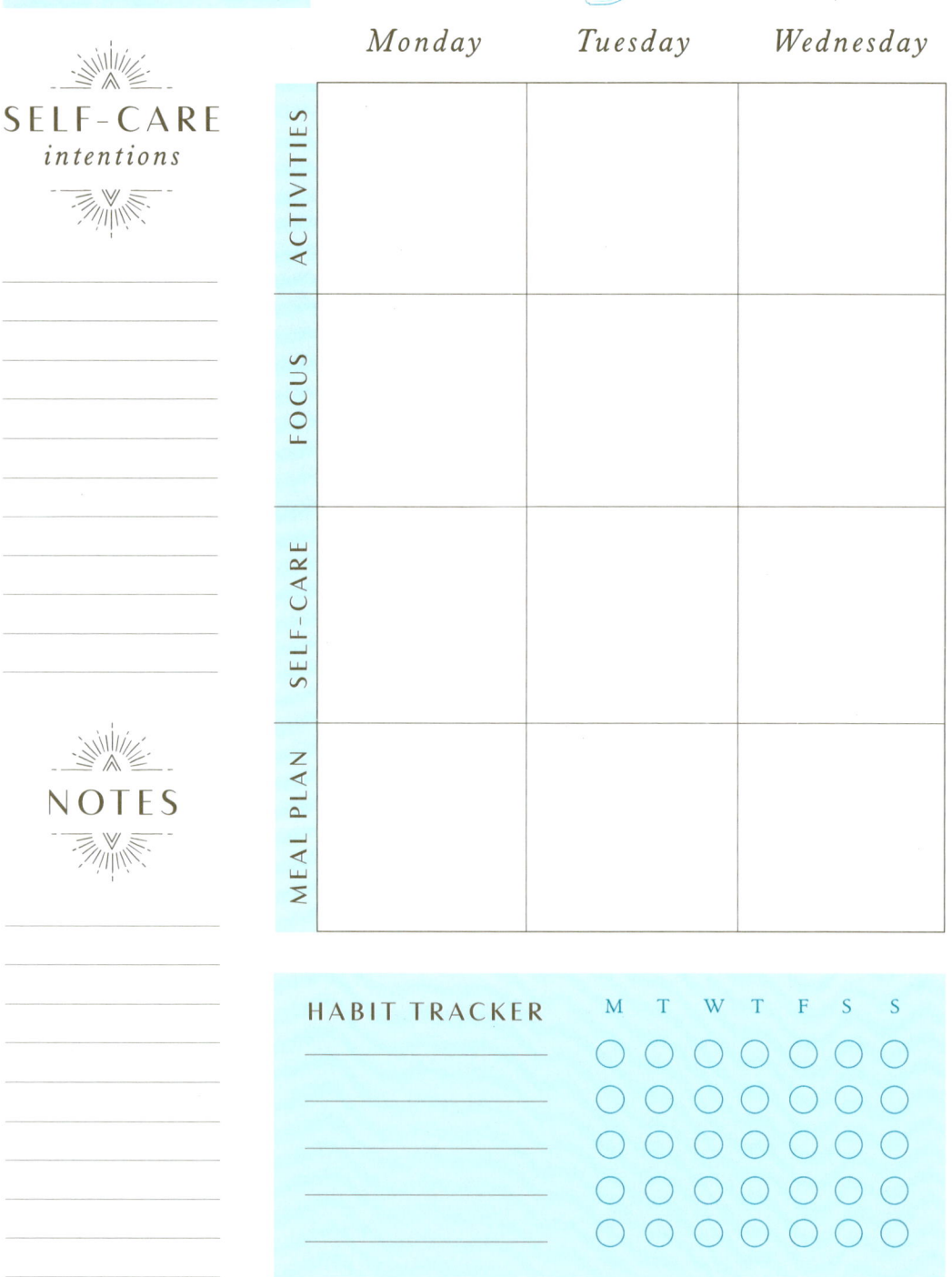

Thursday	Friday	Saturday	Sunday

REFLECTIONS

JOY TO EMBRACE	STRESS TO RELEASE	FOCUSING ON	GRATITUDE FOR

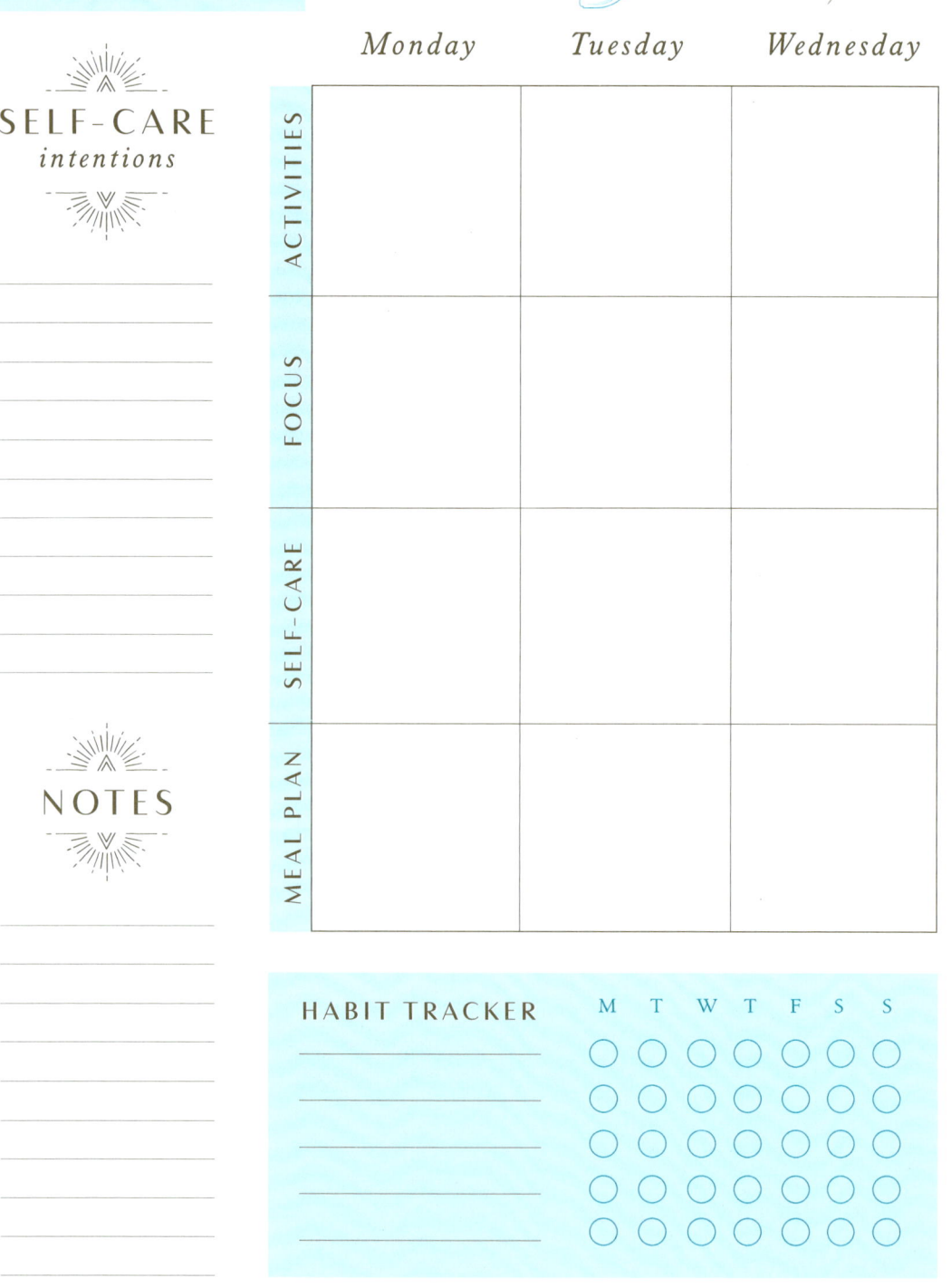

Thursday	Friday	Saturday	Sunday

REFLECTIONS

JOY TO EMBRACE	STRESS TO RELEASE	FOCUSING ON	GRATITUDE FOR

SELF-CARE *intentions*

_____
_____
_____
_____
_____
_____
_____
_____

NOTES

_____
_____
_____
_____
_____
_____
_____
_____

	Monday	Tuesday	Wednesday
ACTIVITIES			
FOCUS			
SELF-CARE			
MEAL PLAN			

HABIT TRACKER

	M	T	W	T	F	S	S
_____	○	○	○	○	○	○	○
_____	○	○	○	○	○	○	○
_____	○	○	○	○	○	○	○
_____	○	○	○	○	○	○	○
_____	○	○	○	○	○	○	○

Thursday	Friday	Saturday	Sunday

REFLECTIONS

JOY TO EMBRACE	STRESS TO RELEASE	FOCUSING ON	GRATITUDE FOR

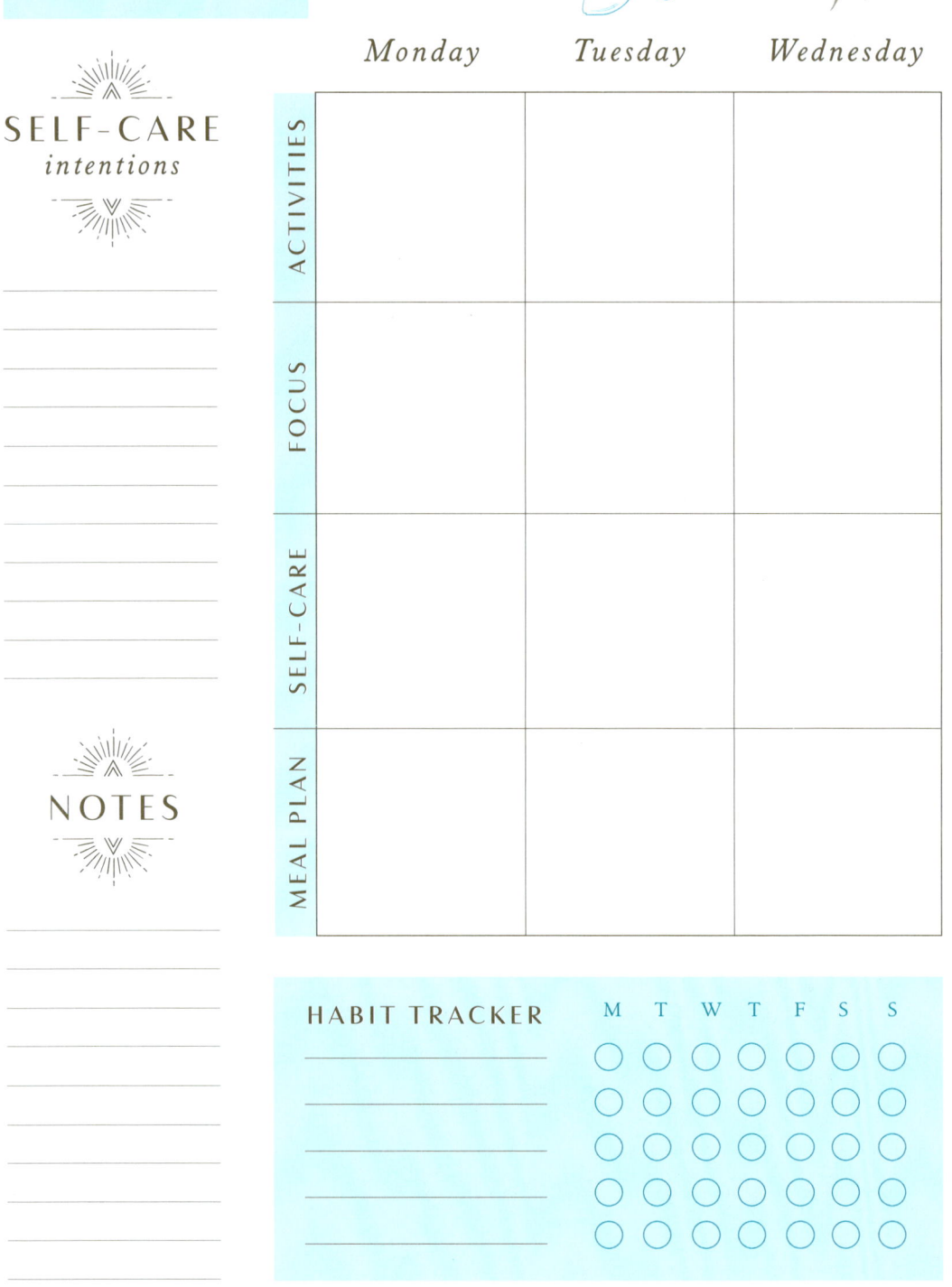

Thursday	Friday	Saturday	Sunday

REFLECTIONS

JOY TO EMBRACE	STRESS TO RELEASE	FOCUSING ON	GRATITUDE FOR

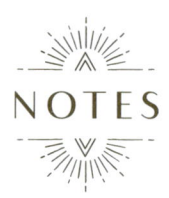

NOTES

"You are imperfect, permanently and inevitably flawed. And you are beautiful."

—AMY BLOOM

SELF-CARE
priorities

	Monday	Tuesday	Wednesday

INSTEAD OF TRYING TO MAKE YOUR LIFE PERFECT, GIVE YOURSELF THE FREEDOM TO MAKE IT AN ADVENTURE, AND GO EVER UPWARD.
–Drew Houston

NOTES

Thursday	Friday	Saturday	Sunday

BIRTHDAYS

SELF-CARE
intentions

	Monday	Tuesday	Wednesday
ACTIVITIES			
FOCUS			
SELF-CARE			
MEAL PLAN			

NOTES

HABIT TRACKER

M T W T F S S

Thursday	Friday	Saturday	Sunday

REFLECTIONS

JOY TO EMBRACE	STRESS TO RELEASE	FOCUSING ON	GRATITUDE FOR

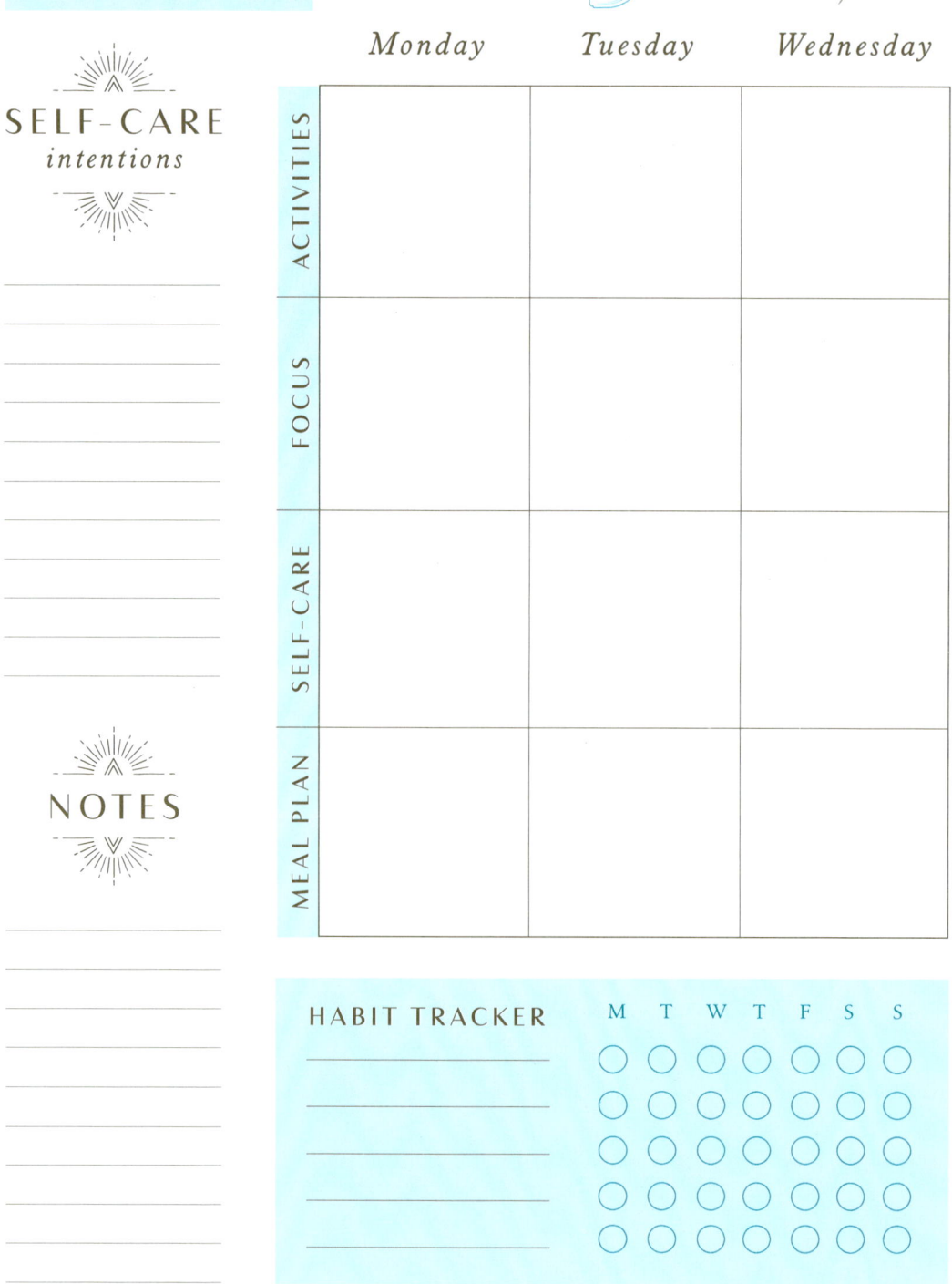

Thursday	Friday	Saturday	Sunday

REFLECTIONS

JOY TO EMBRACE	STRESS TO RELEASE	FOCUSING ON	GRATITUDE FOR

SELF-CARE
intentions

	Monday	Tuesday	Wednesday
ACTIVITIES			
FOCUS			
SELF-CARE			
MEAL PLAN			

NOTES

HABIT TRACKER

M T W T F S S
○ ○ ○ ○ ○ ○ ○
○ ○ ○ ○ ○ ○ ○
○ ○ ○ ○ ○ ○ ○
○ ○ ○ ○ ○ ○ ○
○ ○ ○ ○ ○ ○ ○

Thursday	*Friday*	*Saturday*	*Sunday*

REFLECTIONS

JOY TO EMBRACE	STRESS TO RELEASE	FOCUSING ON	GRATITUDE FOR

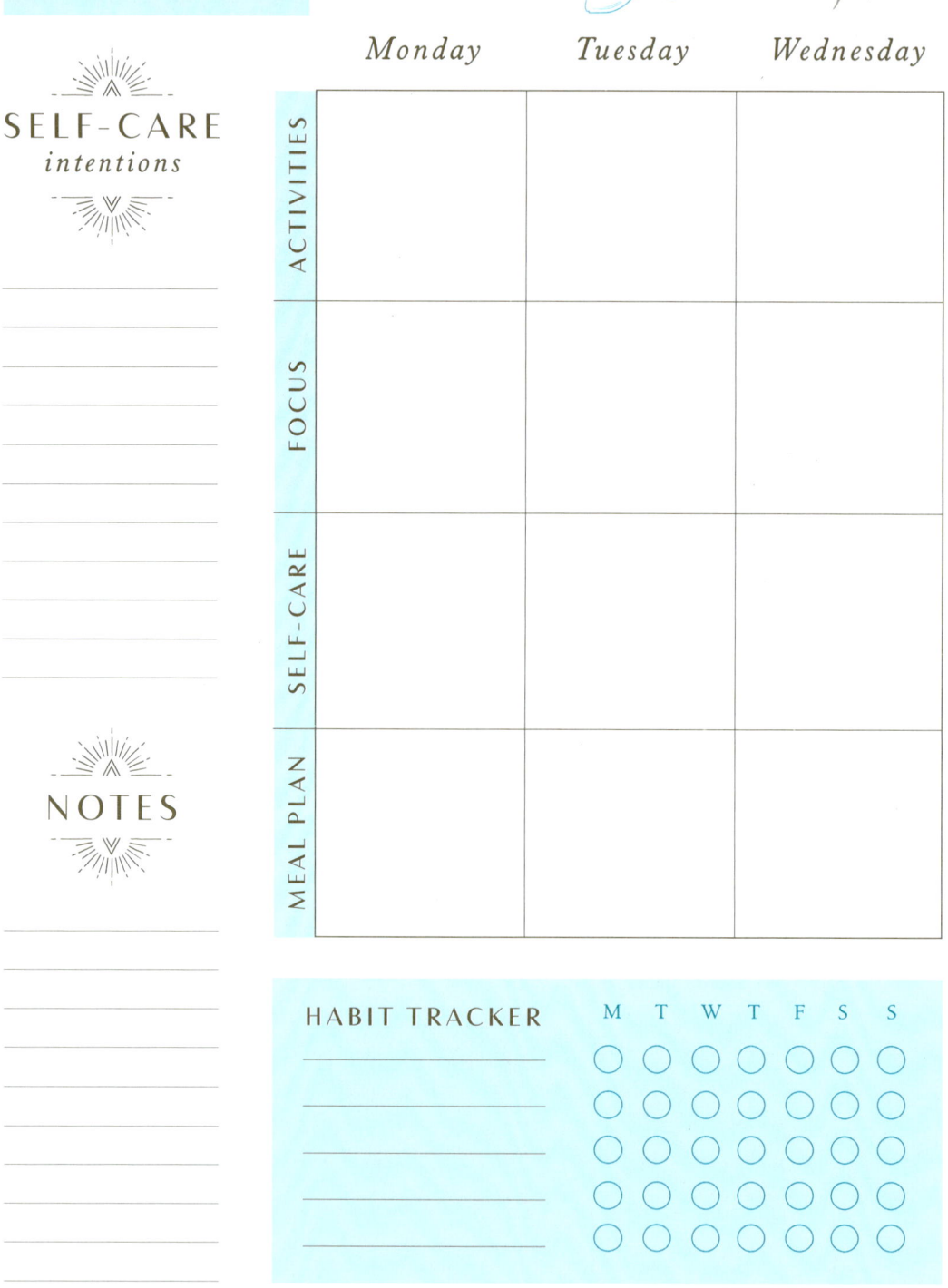

Thursday	Friday	Saturday	Sunday

REFLECTIONS

JOY TO EMBRACE	STRESS TO RELEASE	FOCUSING ON	GRATITUDE FOR

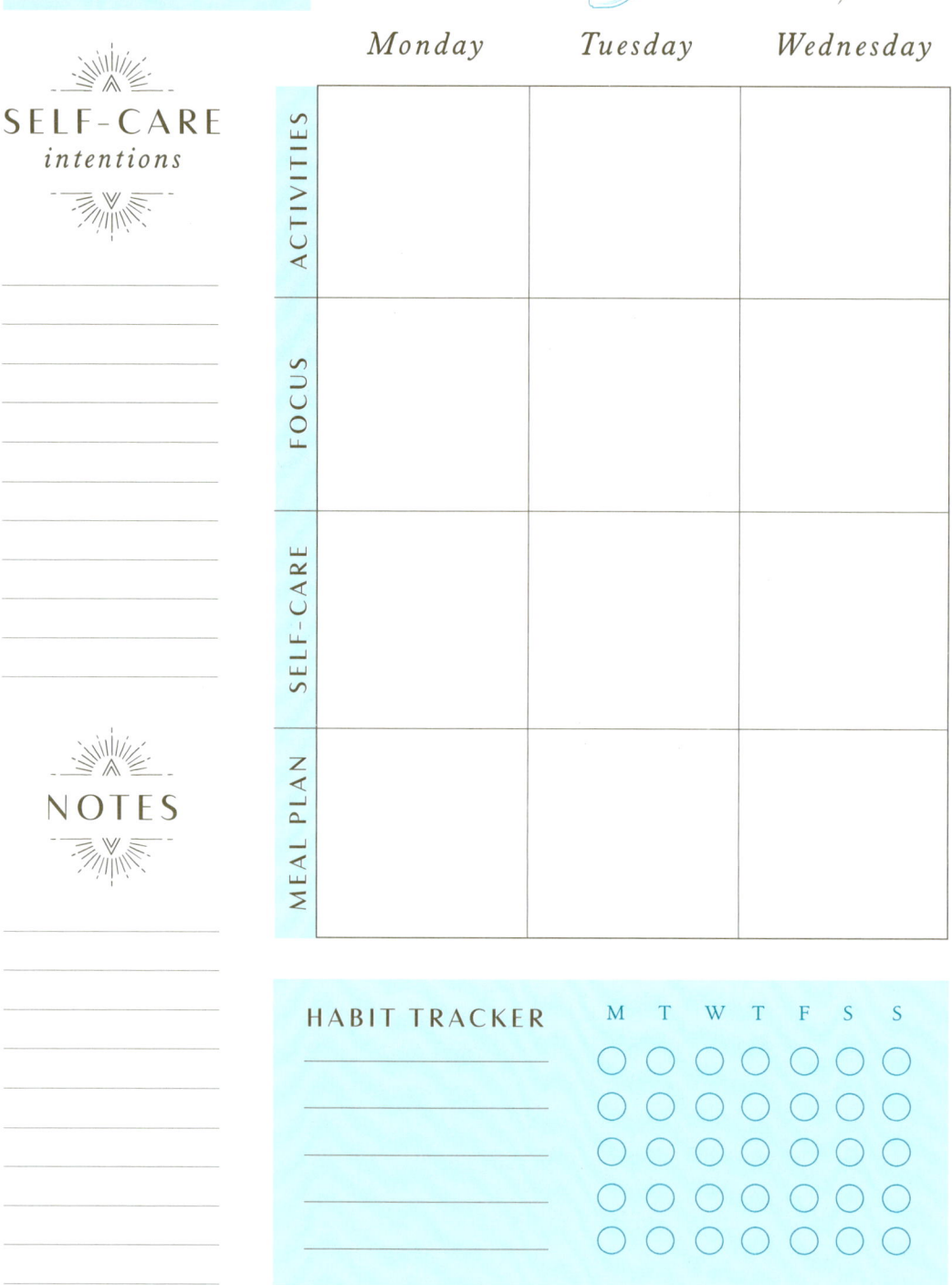

Thursday	Friday	Saturday	Sunday

REFLECTIONS

JOY TO EMBRACE	STRESS TO RELEASE	FOCUSING ON	GRATITUDE FOR

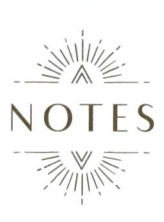

NOTES

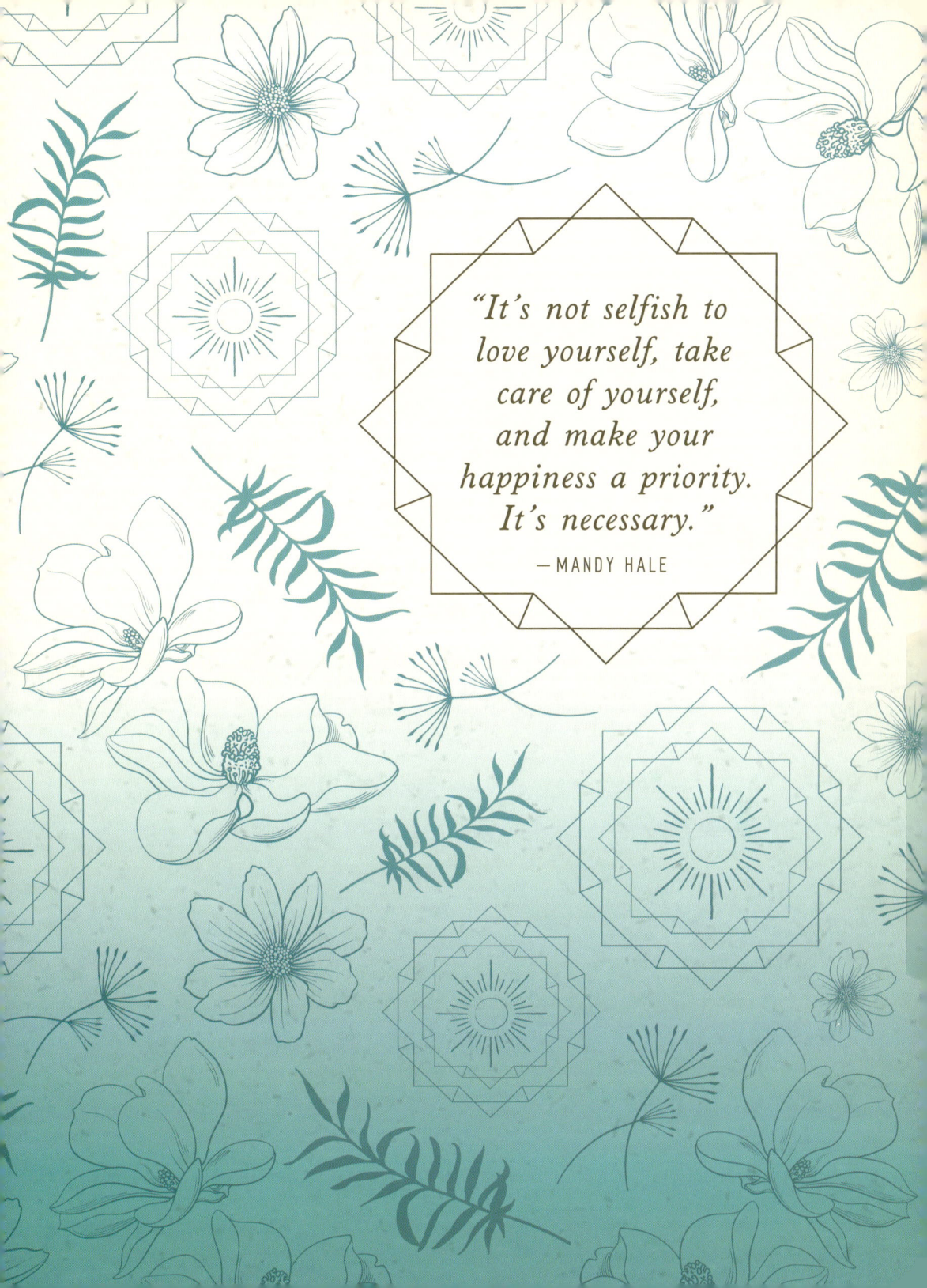

"It's not selfish to love yourself, take care of yourself, and make your happiness a priority. It's necessary."

—MANDY HALE

SELF-CARE
priorities

	Monday	Tuesday	Wednesday

> YOU CAN'T TAKE CARE OF ANYONE ELSE UNLESS YOU FIRST TAKE CARE OF YOURSELF.
> —Michael Hyatt

NOTES

Thursday	Friday	Saturday	Sunday

BIRTHDAYS

SELF-CARE
intentions

	Monday	Tuesday	Wednesday
ACTIVITIES			
FOCUS			
SELF-CARE			
MEAL PLAN			

NOTES

HABIT TRACKER

M T W T F S S

Thursday	Friday	Saturday	Sunday

REFLECTIONS

JOY TO EMBRACE	STRESS TO RELEASE	FOCUSING ON	GRATITUDE FOR

SELF-CARE
intentions

	Monday	Tuesday	Wednesday
ACTIVITIES			
FOCUS			
SELF-CARE			
MEAL PLAN			

NOTES

HABIT TRACKER

M T W T F S S

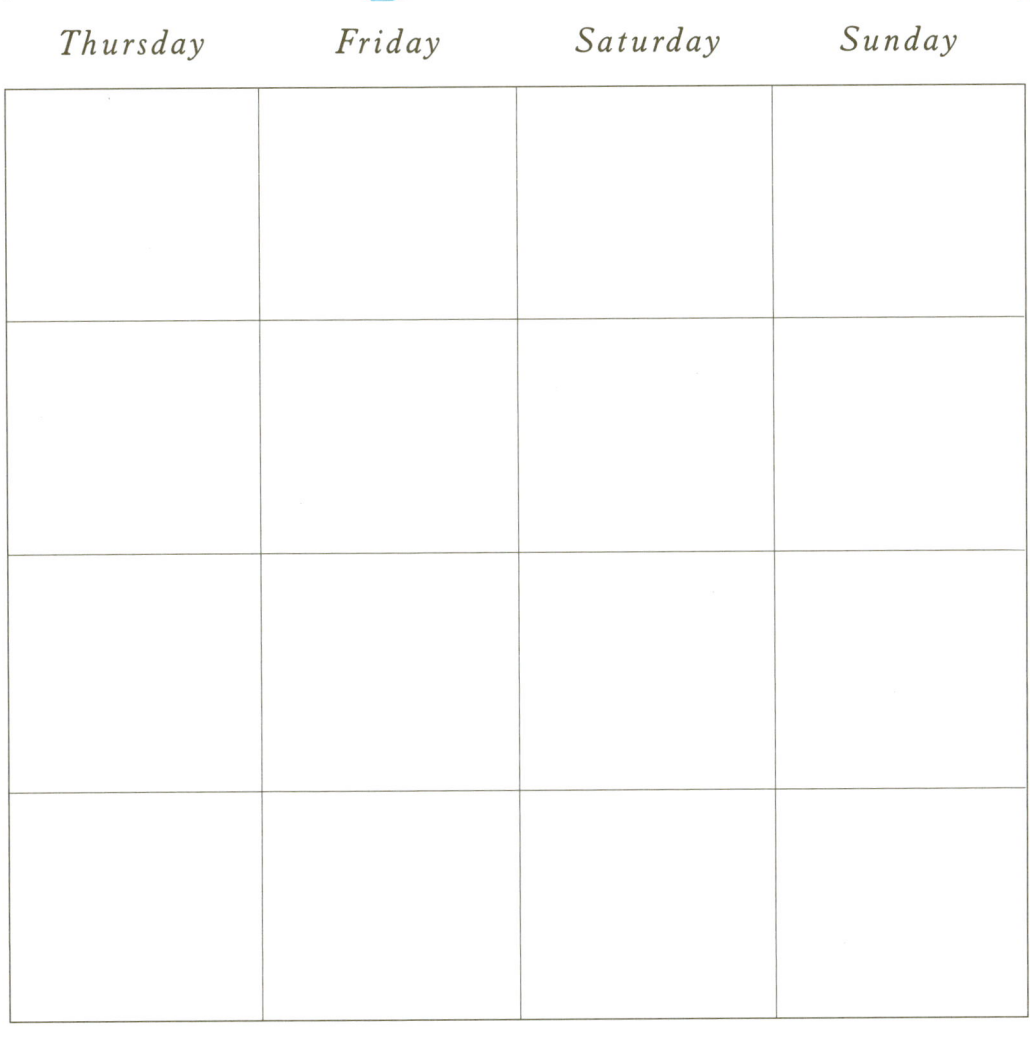

Thursday	Friday	Saturday	Sunday

REFLECTIONS

JOY TO EMBRACE	STRESS TO RELEASE	FOCUSING ON	GRATITUDE FOR

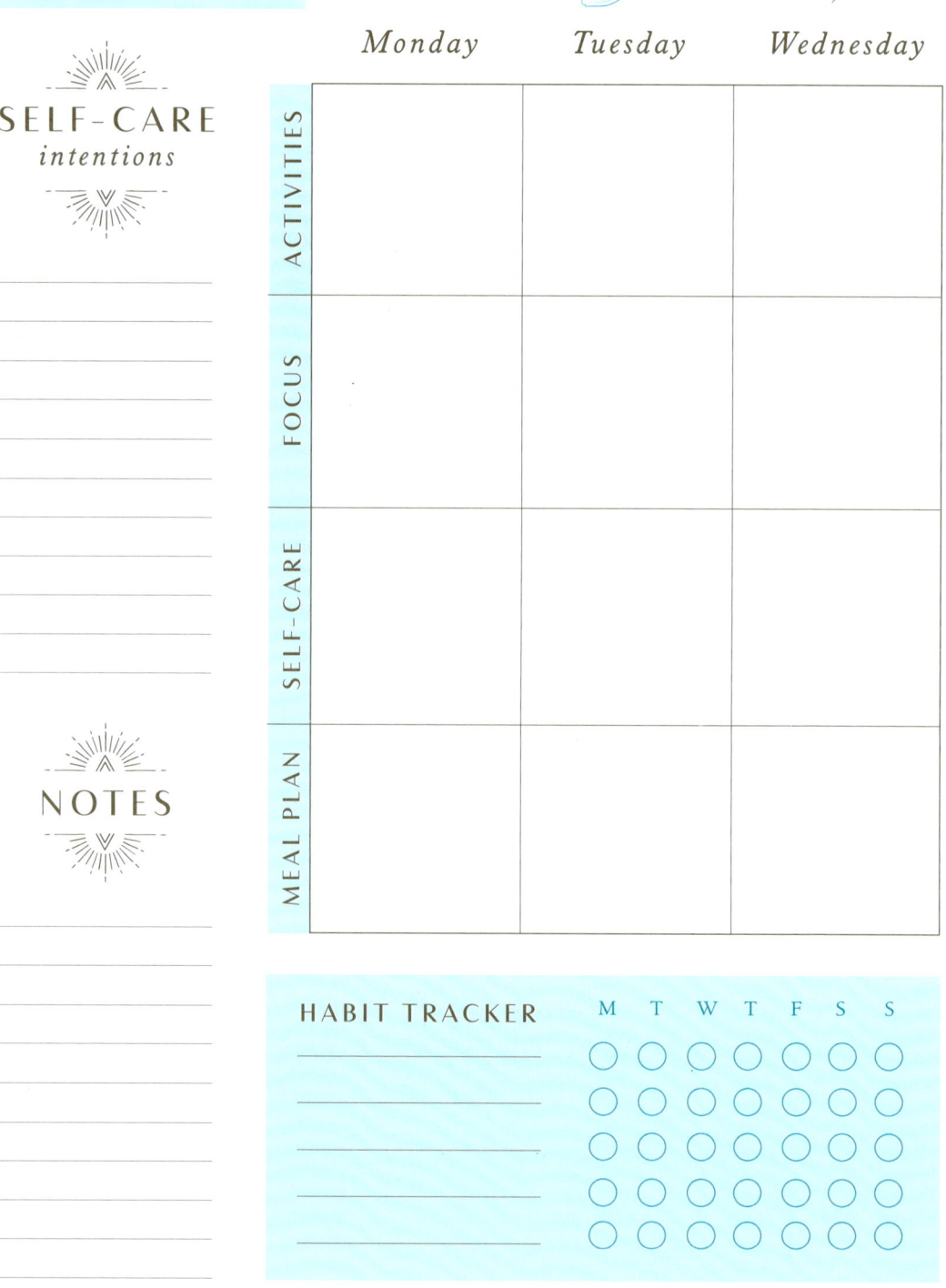

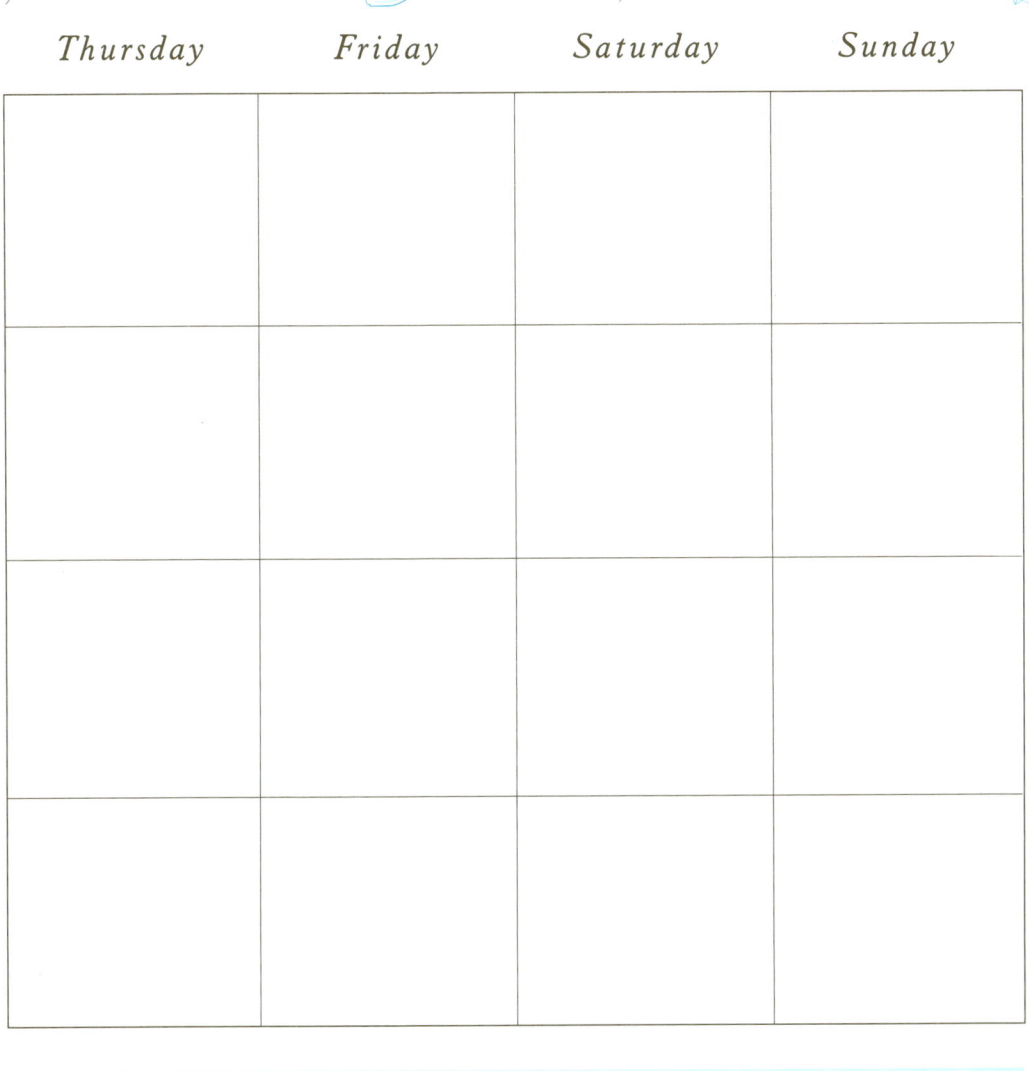

Thursday	Friday	Saturday	Sunday

REFLECTIONS

JOY TO EMBRACE	STRESS TO RELEASE	FOCUSING ON	GRATITUDE FOR

SELF-CARE
intentions

	Monday	Tuesday	Wednesday
ACTIVITIES			
FOCUS			
SELF-CARE			
MEAL PLAN			

NOTES

HABIT TRACKER   M T W T F S S

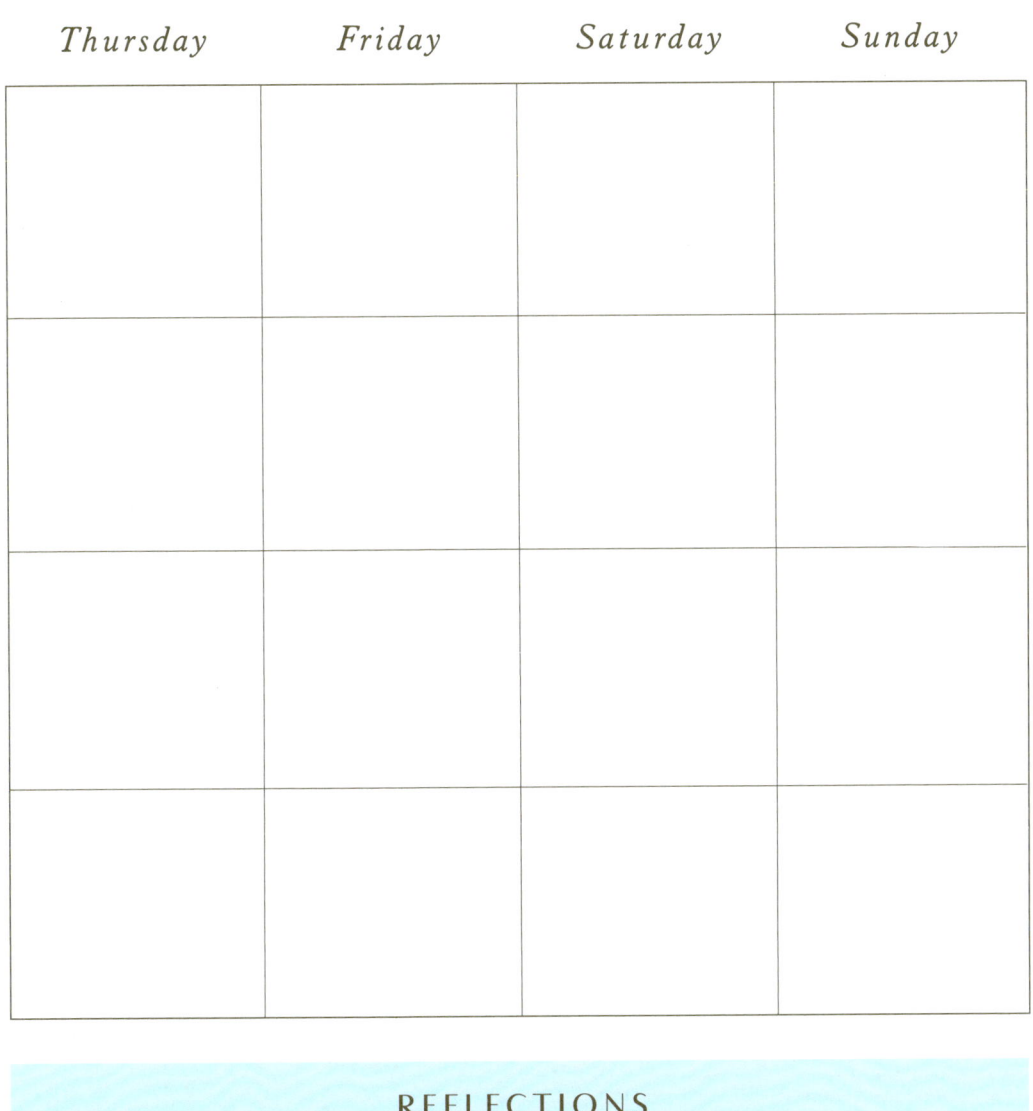

Thursday	Friday	Saturday	Sunday

REFLECTIONS

JOY TO EMBRACE	STRESS TO RELEASE	FOCUSING ON	GRATITUDE FOR

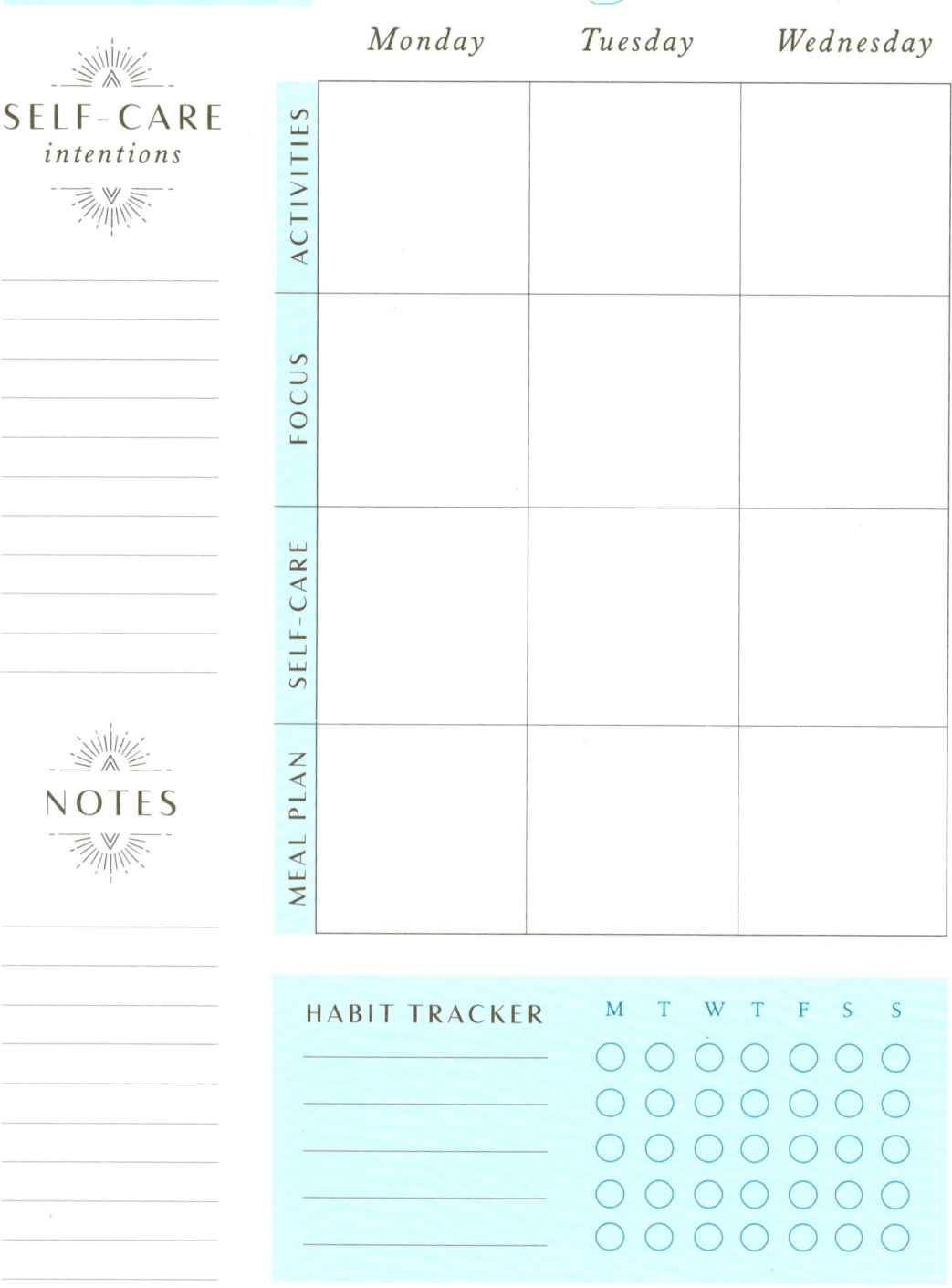

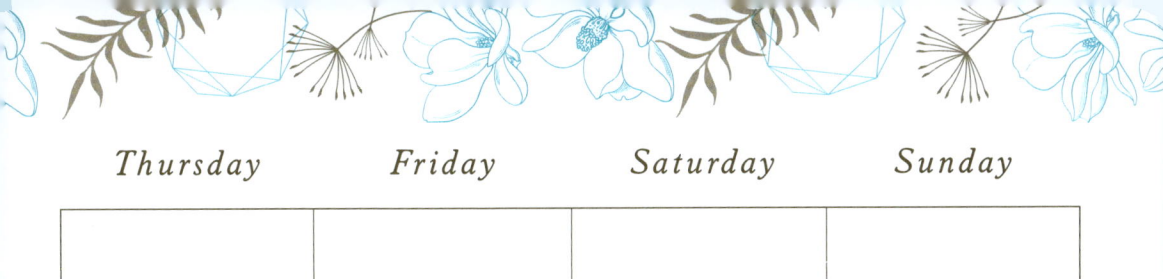

Thursday	Friday	Saturday	Sunday

REFLECTIONS

JOY TO EMBRACE	STRESS TO RELEASE	FOCUSING ON	GRATITUDE FOR

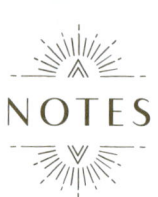

NOTES

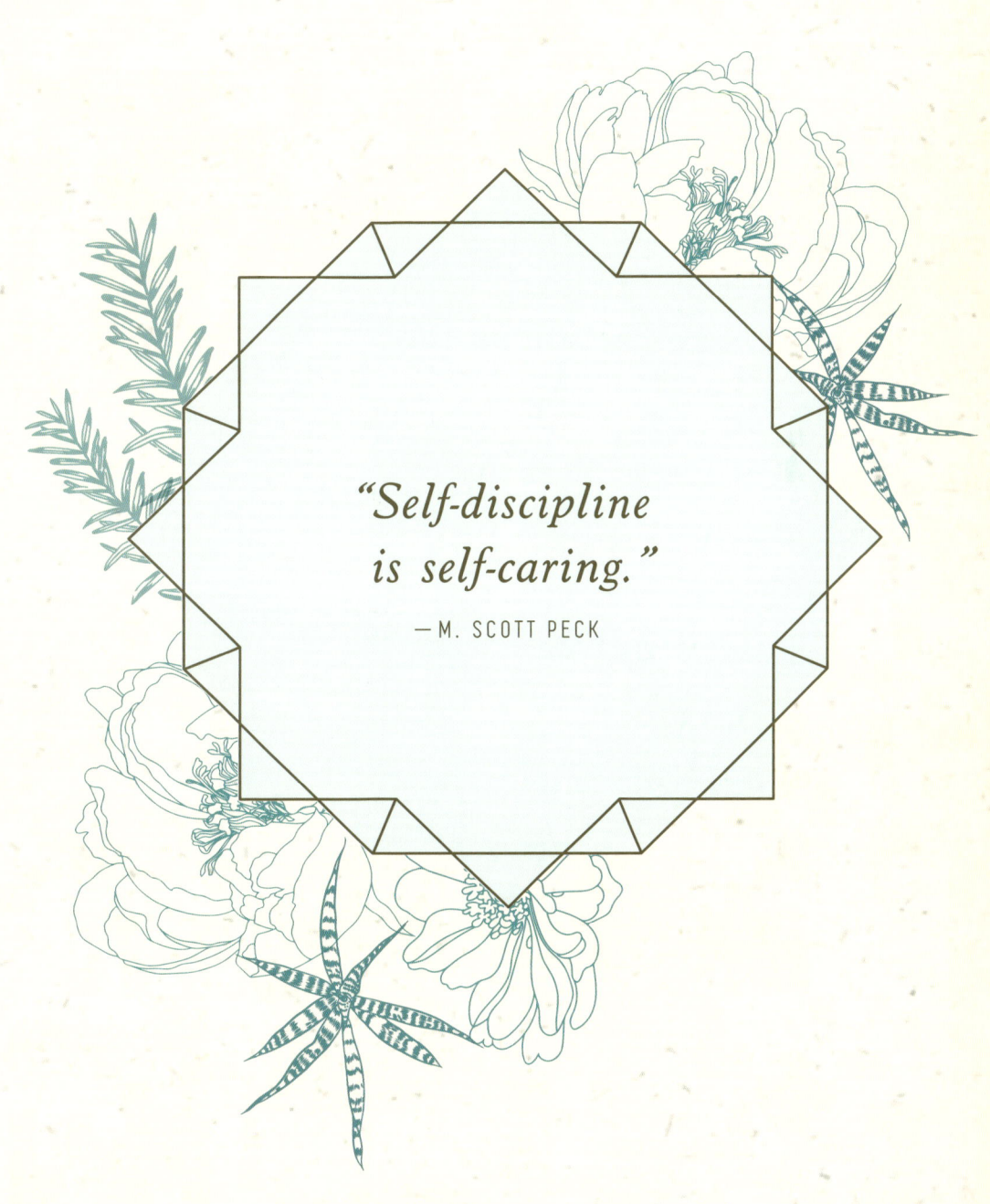

"Self-discipline is self-caring."
—M. SCOTT PECK

SELF-CARE
priorities

	Monday	Tuesday	Wednesday

EVERY ACT OF SELF-CARE IS A POWERFUL DECLARATION: I AM ON MY SIDE; I AM ON MY SIDE; EACH DAY I AM MORE AND MORE ON MY OWN SIDE.
—Susan Weiss Berry

NOTES

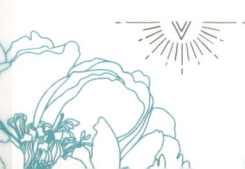

Thursday	Friday	Saturday	Sunday

BIRTHDAYS

SELF-CARE
intentions

	Monday	Tuesday	Wednesday
ACTIVITIES			
FOCUS			
SELF-CARE			
MEAL PLAN			

NOTES

HABIT TRACKER

M T W T F S S
○ ○ ○ ○ ○ ○ ○
○ ○ ○ ○ ○ ○ ○
○ ○ ○ ○ ○ ○ ○
○ ○ ○ ○ ○ ○ ○
○ ○ ○ ○ ○ ○ ○

Thursday	Friday	Saturday	Sunday

REFLECTIONS

JOY TO EMBRACE	STRESS TO RELEASE	FOCUSING ON	GRATITUDE FOR

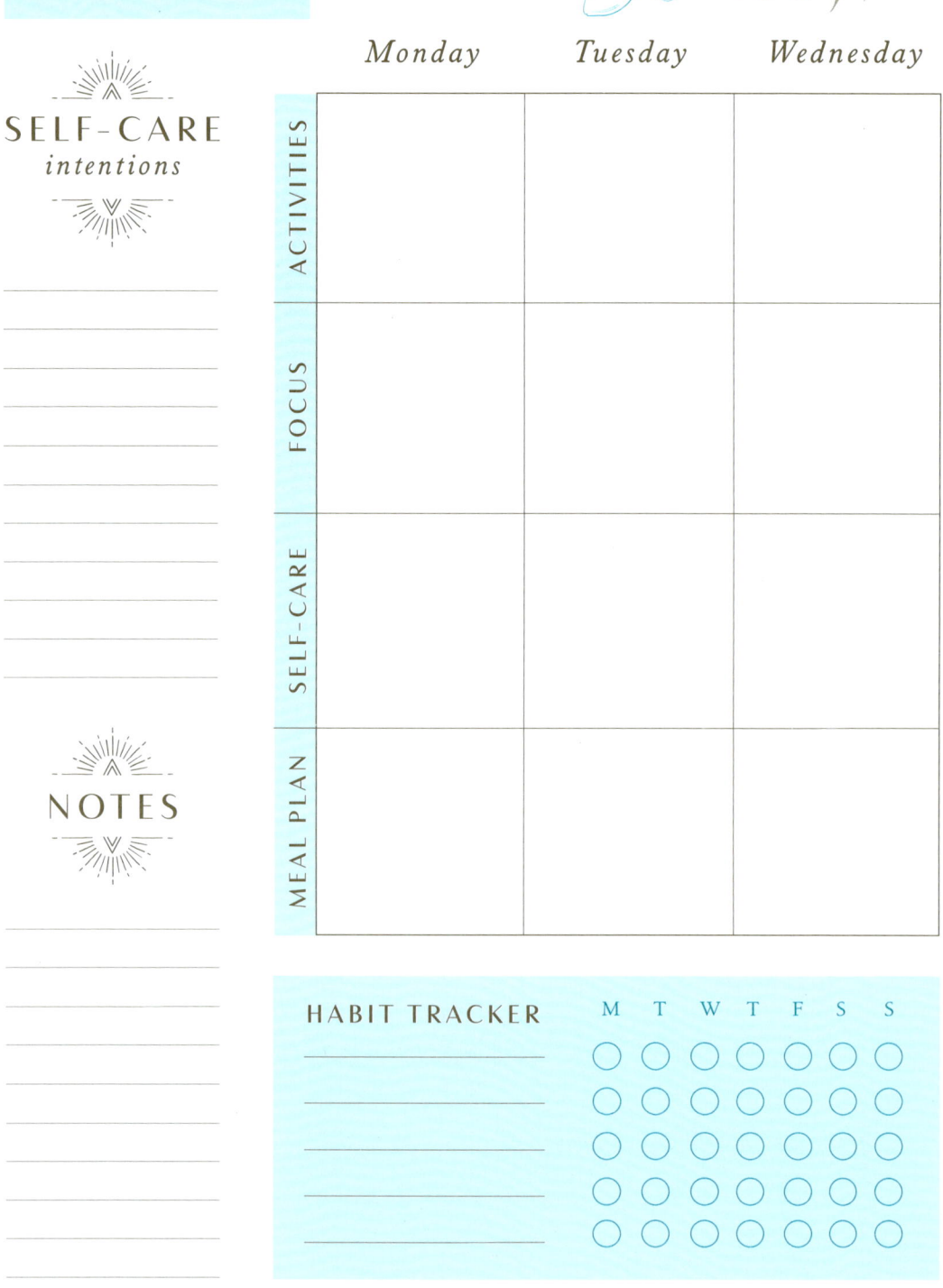

Thursday	Friday	Saturday	Sunday

REFLECTIONS

JOY TO EMBRACE	STRESS TO RELEASE	FOCUSING ON	GRATITUDE FOR

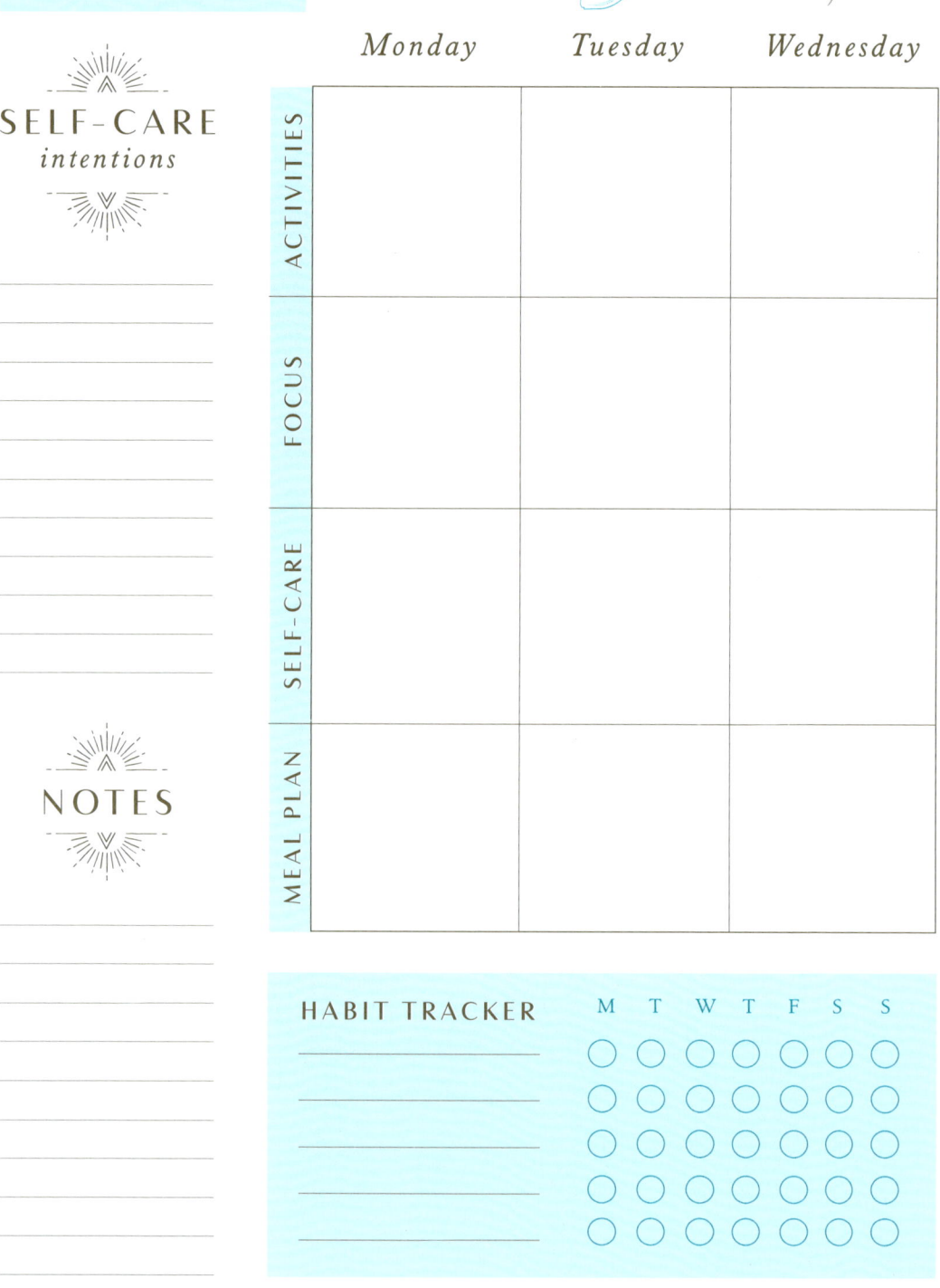

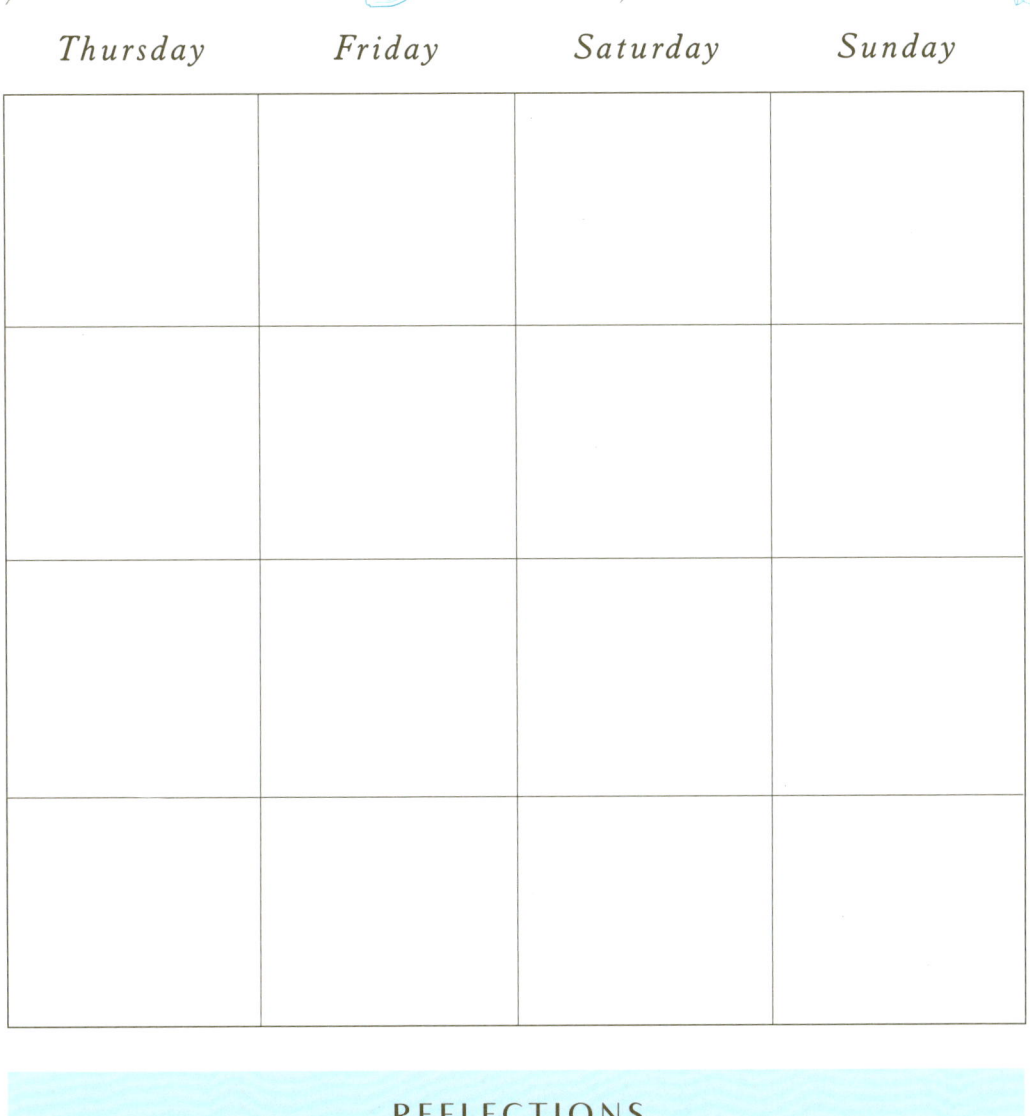

Thursday	Friday	Saturday	Sunday

REFLECTIONS

JOY TO EMBRACE	STRESS TO RELEASE	FOCUSING ON	GRATITUDE FOR

SELF-CARE
intentions

	Monday	Tuesday	Wednesday
ACTIVITIES			
FOCUS			
SELF-CARE			
MEAL PLAN			

NOTES

HABIT TRACKER M T W T F S S

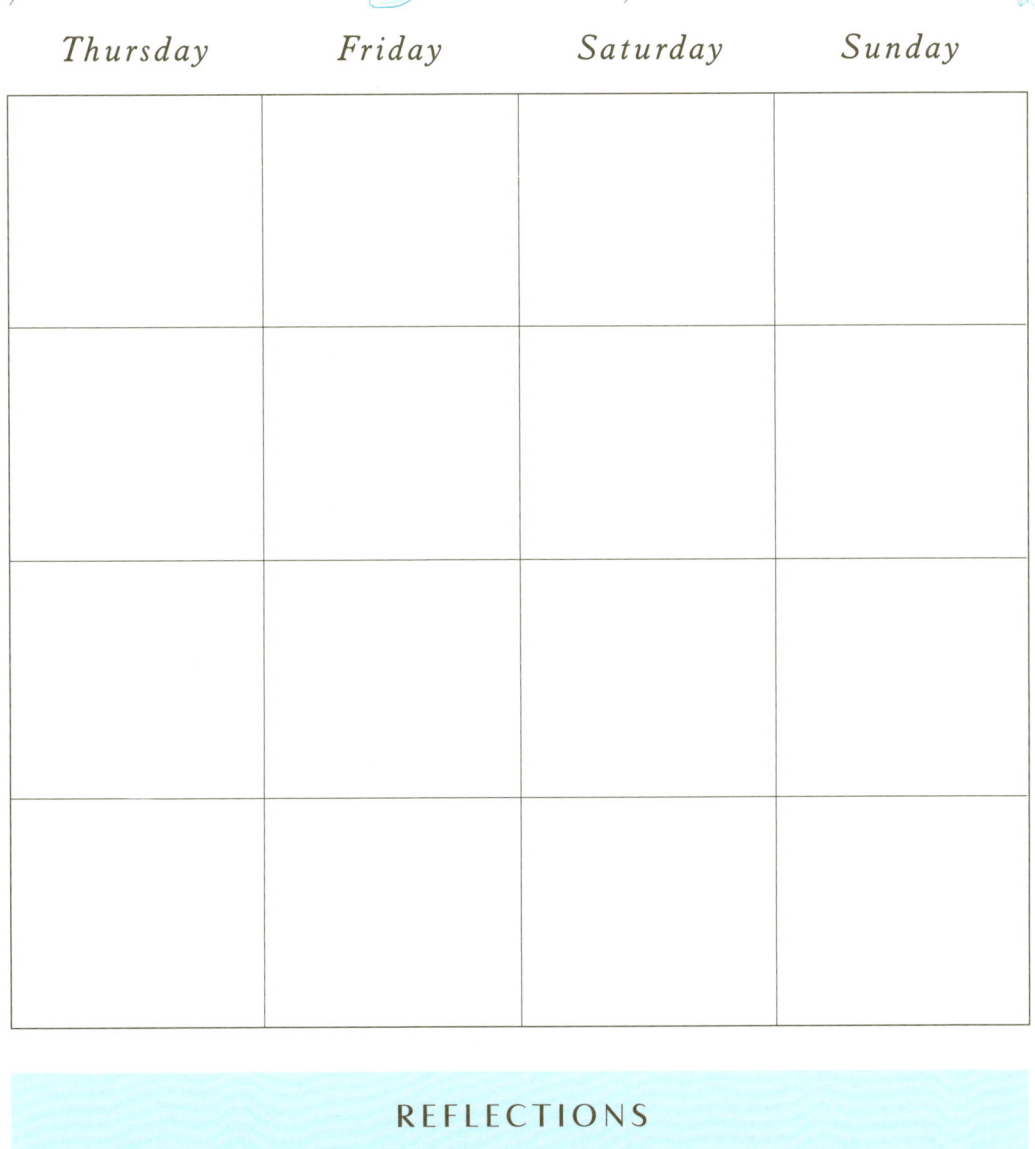

Thursday	Friday	Saturday	Sunday

REFLECTIONS

JOY TO EMBRACE	STRESS TO RELEASE	FOCUSING ON	GRATITUDE FOR

SELF-CARE
intentions

NOTES

	Monday	Tuesday	Wednesday
ACTIVITIES			
FOCUS			
SELF-CARE			
MEAL PLAN			

HABIT TRACKER

M T W T F S S

Thursday	Friday	Saturday	Sunday

REFLECTIONS

JOY TO EMBRACE	STRESS TO RELEASE	FOCUSING ON	GRATITUDE FOR

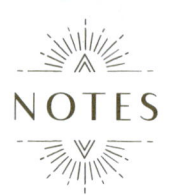

NOTES

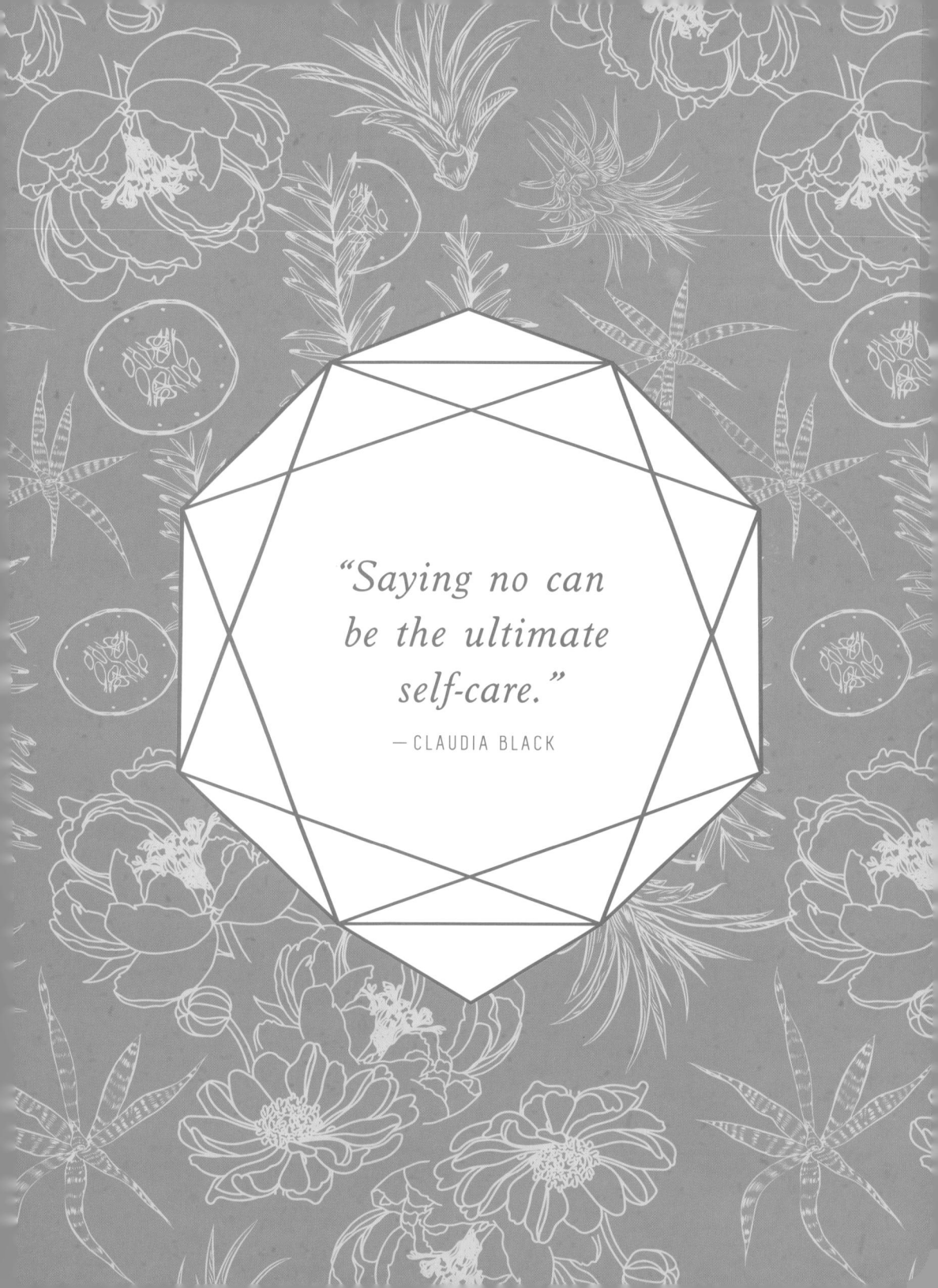

SELF-CARE
priorities

	Monday	Tuesday	Wednesday

> LOVE YOURSELF ENOUGH TO SET BOUNDARIES. YOUR TIME AND ENERGY ARE PRECIOUS. YOU GET TO CHOOSE HOW YOU USE IT.
> —Anna Taylor

NOTES

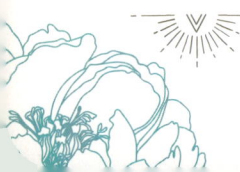

Thursday	Friday	Saturday	Sunday

BIRTHDAYS

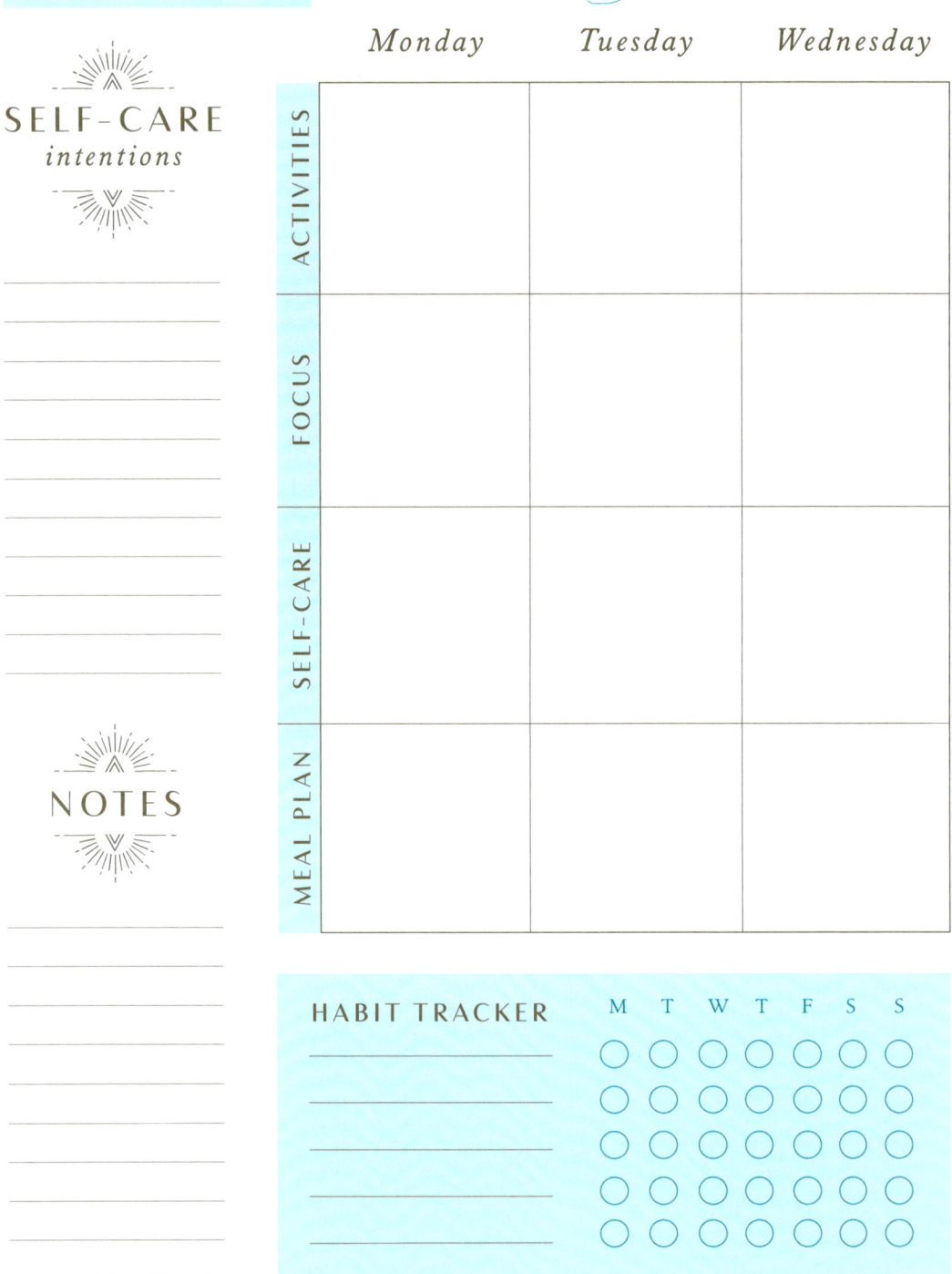

Thursday	Friday	Saturday	Sunday

REFLECTIONS

JOY TO EMBRACE	STRESS TO RELEASE	FOCUSING ON	GRATITUDE FOR

SELF-CARE
intentions

	Monday	Tuesday	Wednesday
ACTIVITIES			
FOCUS			
SELF-CARE			
MEAL PLAN			

NOTES

HABIT TRACKER

M T W T F S S

Thursday	*Friday*	*Saturday*	*Sunday*

REFLECTIONS

JOY TO EMBRACE	STRESS TO RELEASE	FOCUSING ON	GRATITUDE FOR

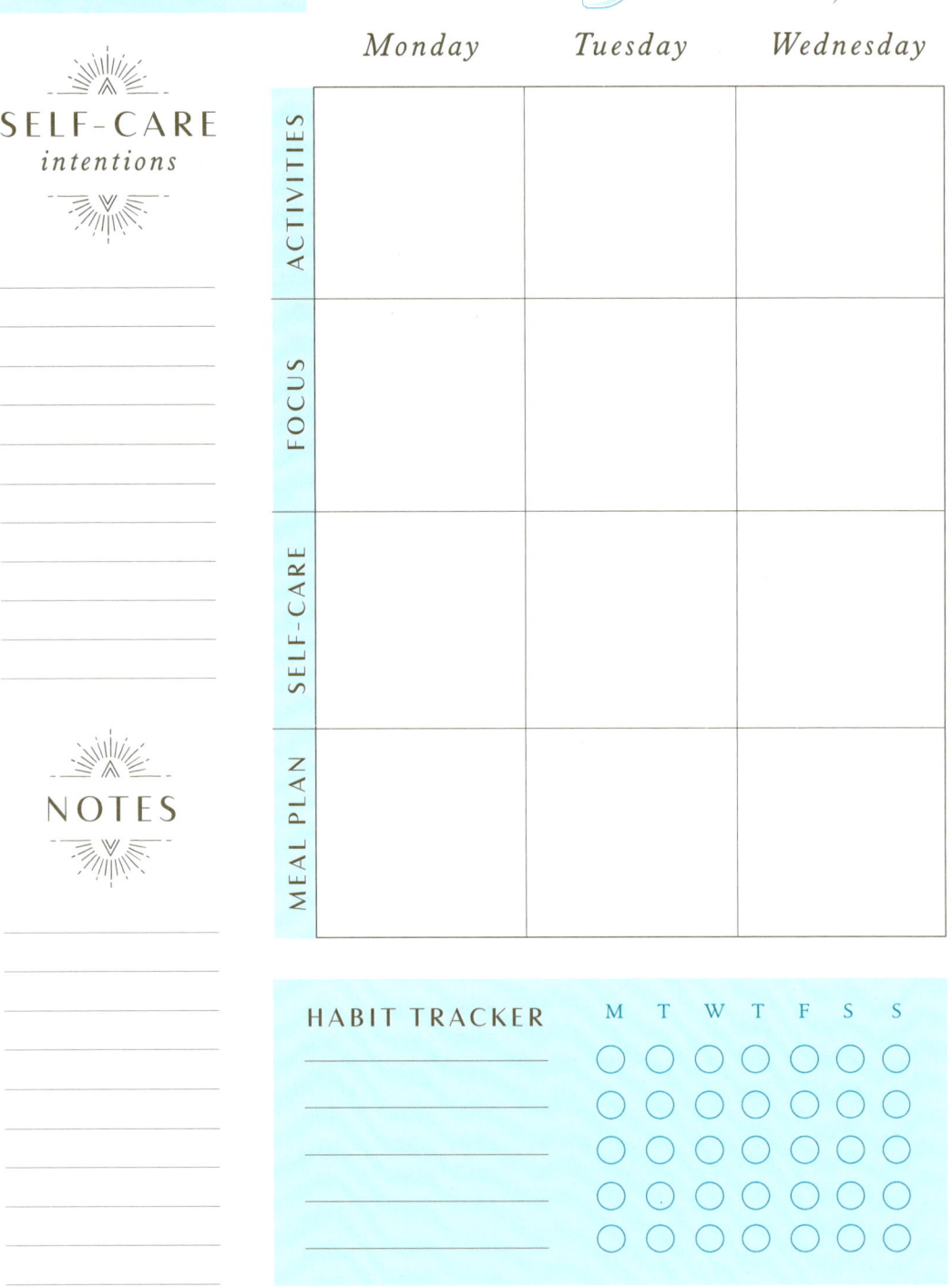

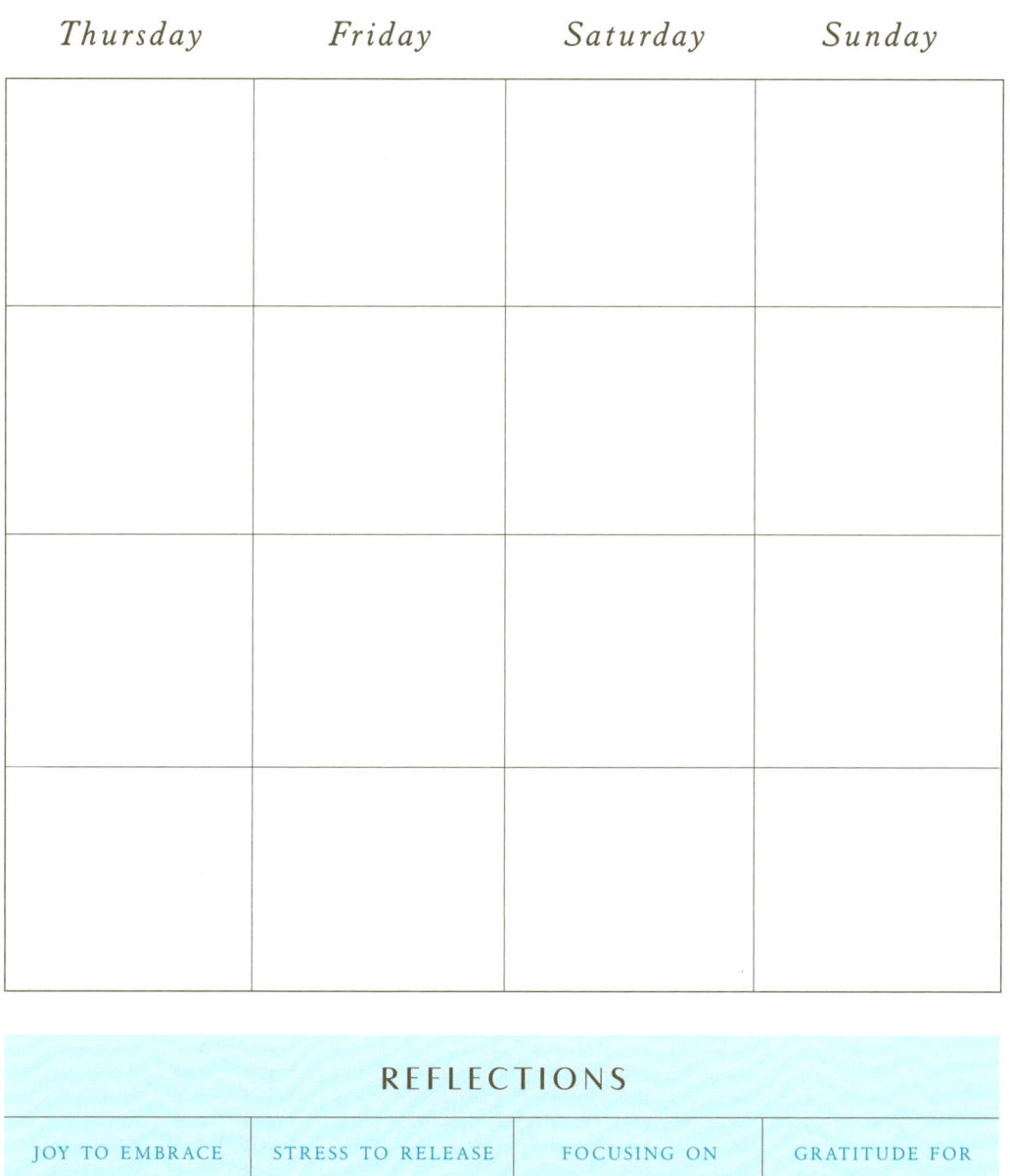

Thursday	Friday	Saturday	Sunday

REFLECTIONS

JOY TO EMBRACE	STRESS TO RELEASE	FOCUSING ON	GRATITUDE FOR

SELF-CARE
intentions

	Monday	Tuesday	Wednesday
ACTIVITIES			
FOCUS			
SELF-CARE			
MEAL PLAN			

NOTES

HABIT TRACKER

	M	T	W	T	F	S	S
_____	○	○	○	○	○	○	○
_____	○	○	○	○	○	○	○
_____	○	○	○	○	○	○	○
_____	○	○	○	○	○	○	○
_____	○	○	○	○	○	○	○

Thursday	Friday	Saturday	Sunday

REFLECTIONS

JOY TO EMBRACE	STRESS TO RELEASE	FOCUSING ON	GRATITUDE FOR

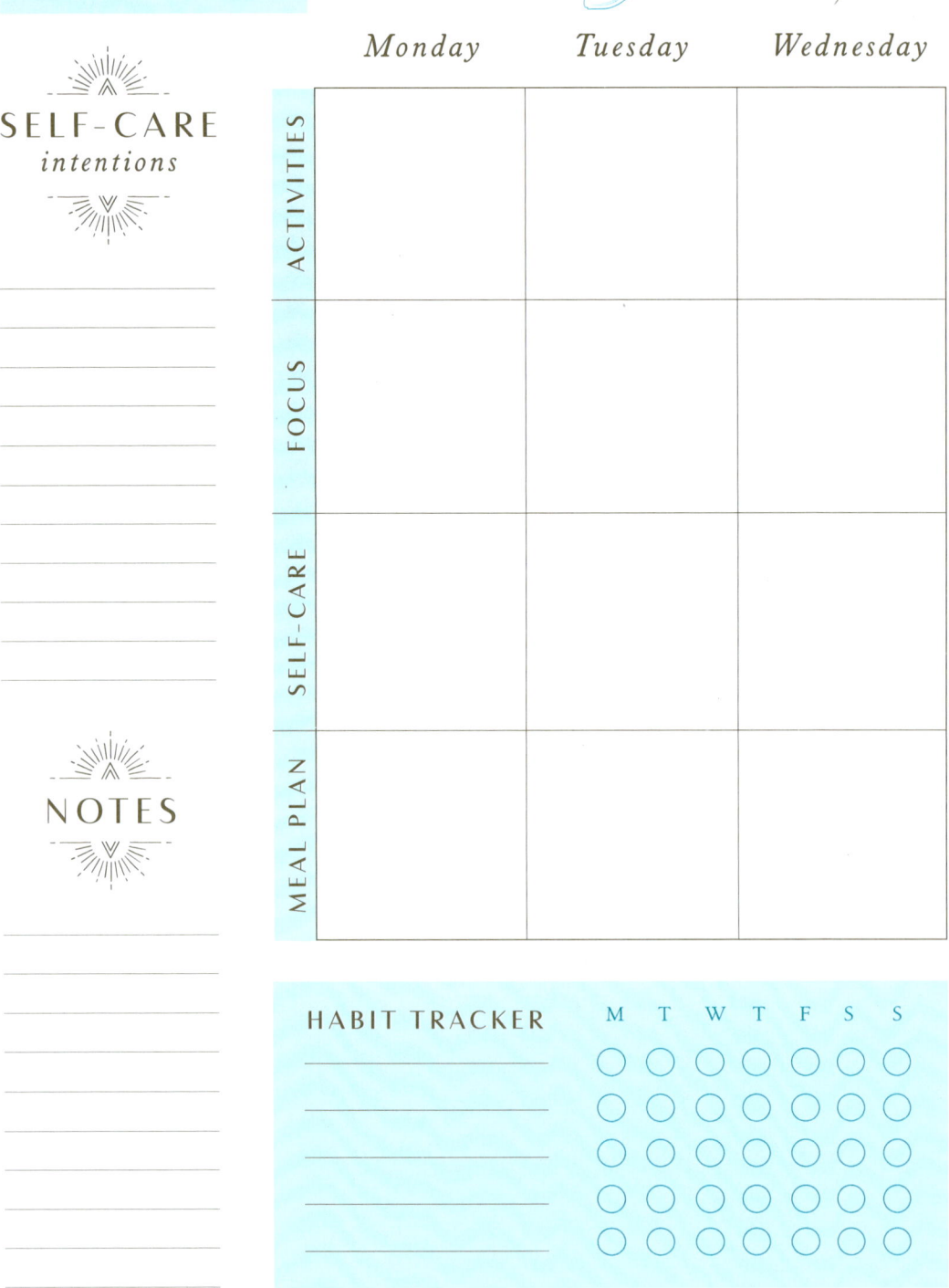

Thursday	Friday	Saturday	Sunday

REFLECTIONS

JOY TO EMBRACE	STRESS TO RELEASE	FOCUSING ON	GRATITUDE FOR

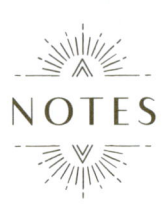

NOTES

"Acknowledge, accept, and honor that you deserve your own deepest compassion and love."

— NANETTE MATHEWS

SELF-CARE
priorities

	Monday	Tuesday	Wednesday

> THE LOVE AND ATTENTION YOU ALWAYS THOUGHT YOU WANTED FROM SOMEONE ELSE IS THE LOVE AND ATTENTION YOU FIRST NEED TO GIVE TO YOURSELF.
> —*Bryant McGill*

NOTES

Thursday	Friday	Saturday	Sunday

BIRTHDAYS

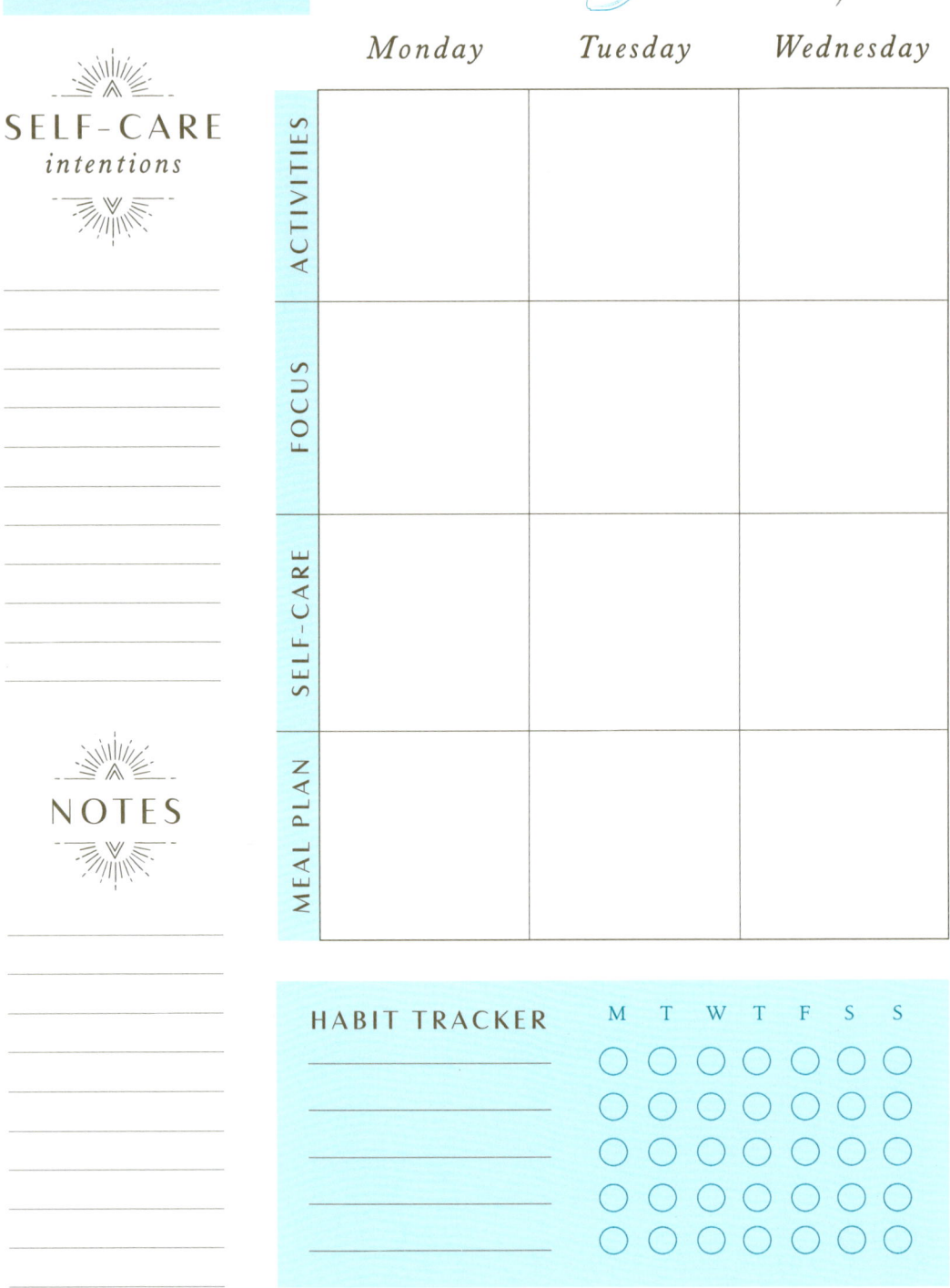

Thursday	Friday	Saturday	Sunday

REFLECTIONS

JOY TO EMBRACE	STRESS TO RELEASE	FOCUSING ON	GRATITUDE FOR

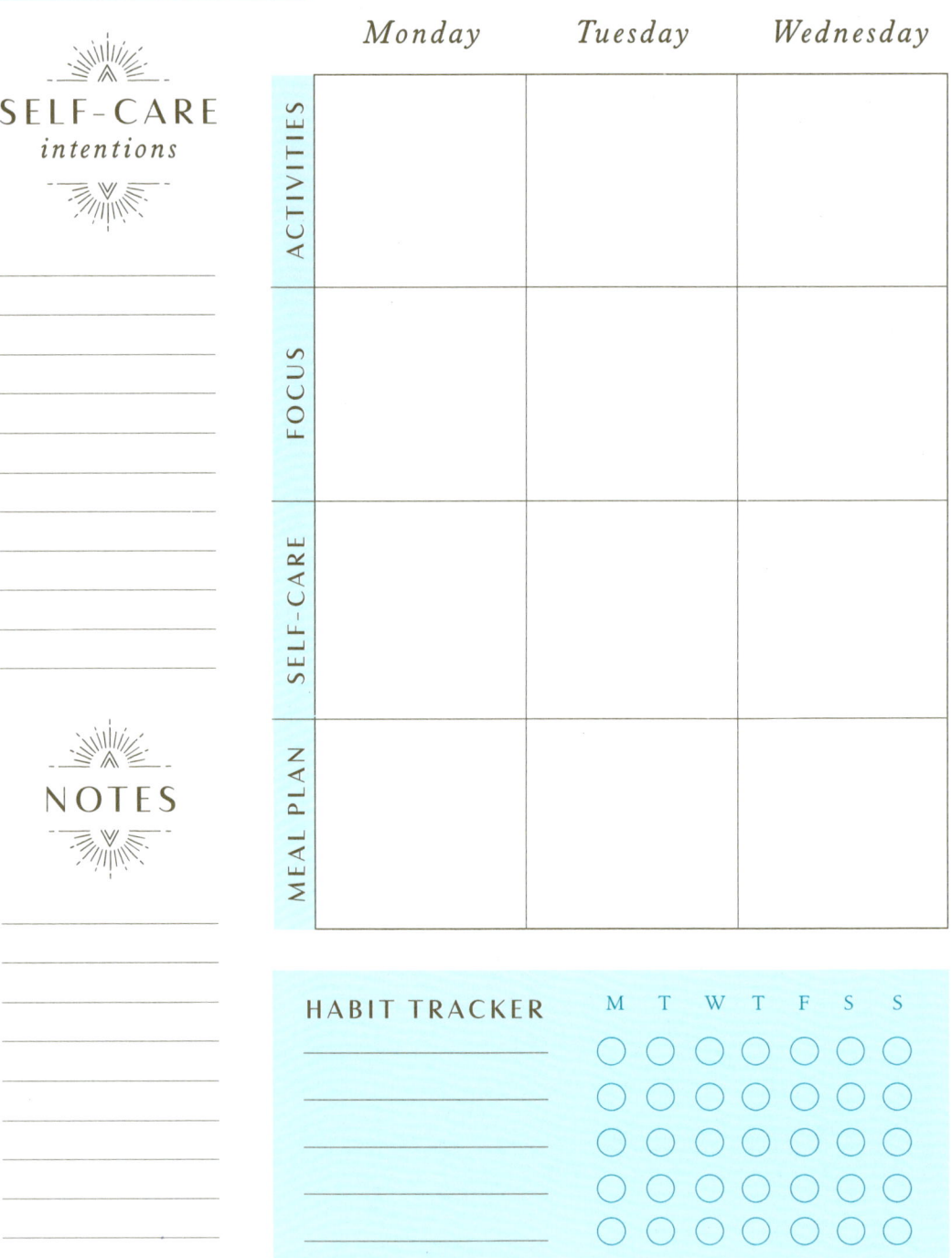

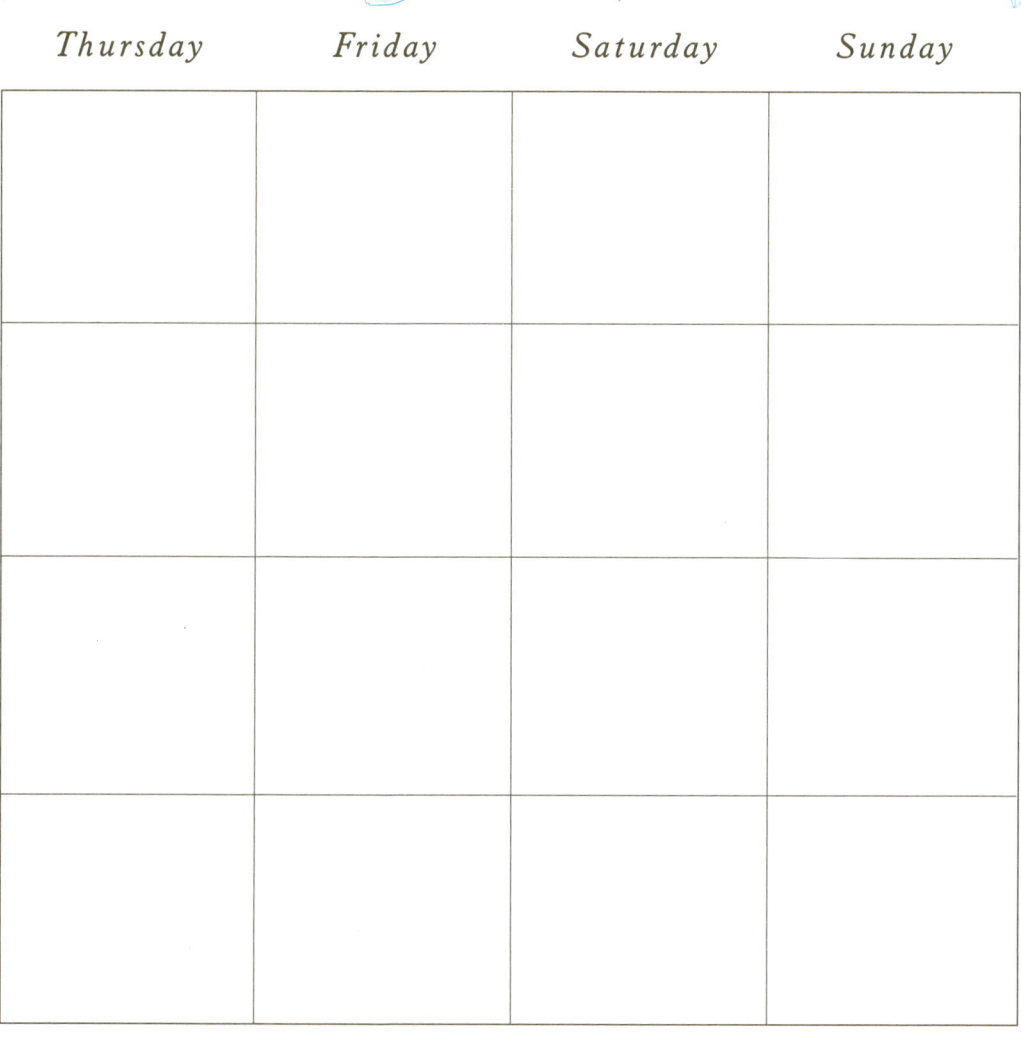

Thursday	Friday	Saturday	Sunday

REFLECTIONS

JOY TO EMBRACE	STRESS TO RELEASE	FOCUSING ON	GRATITUDE FOR

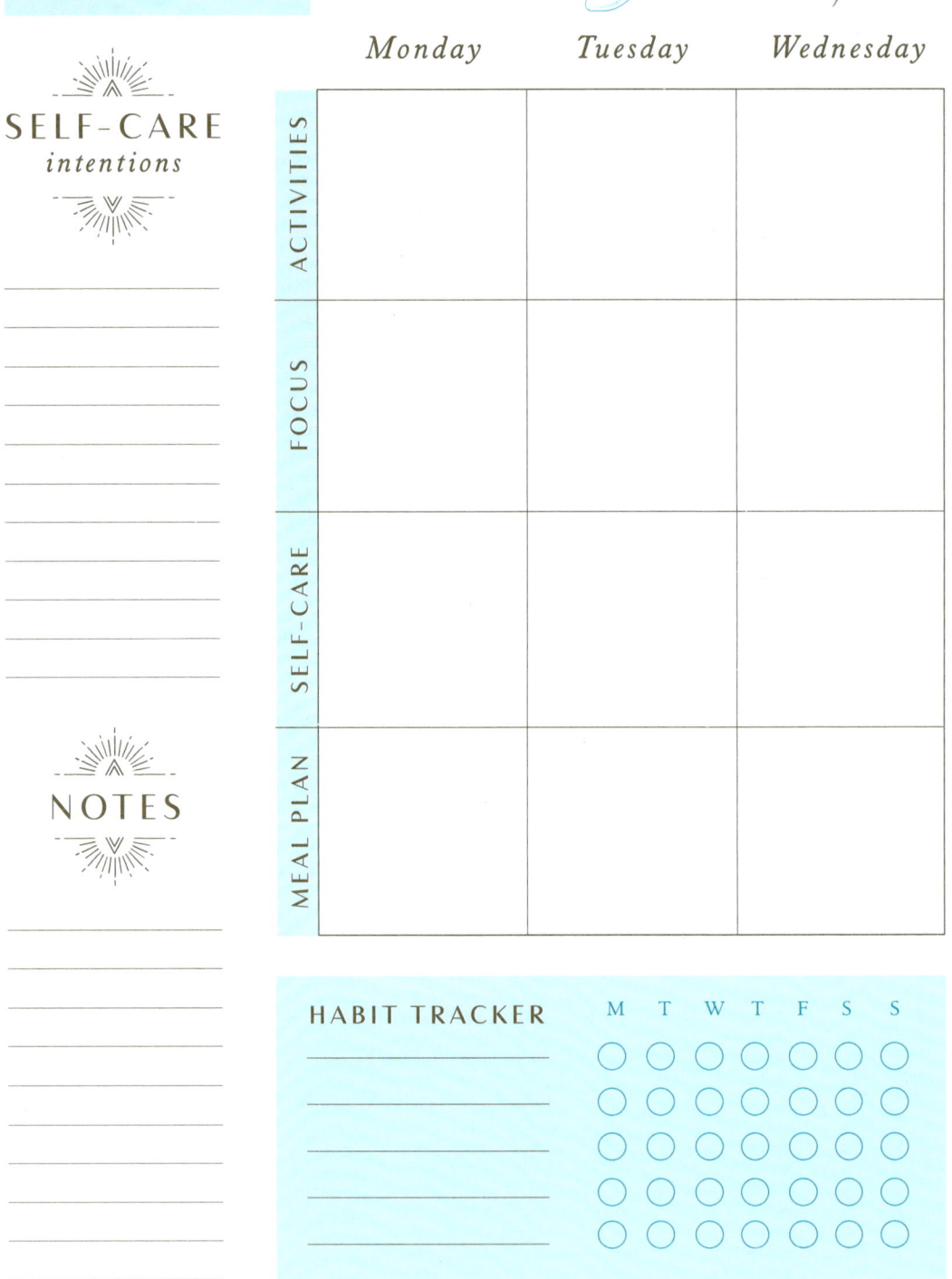

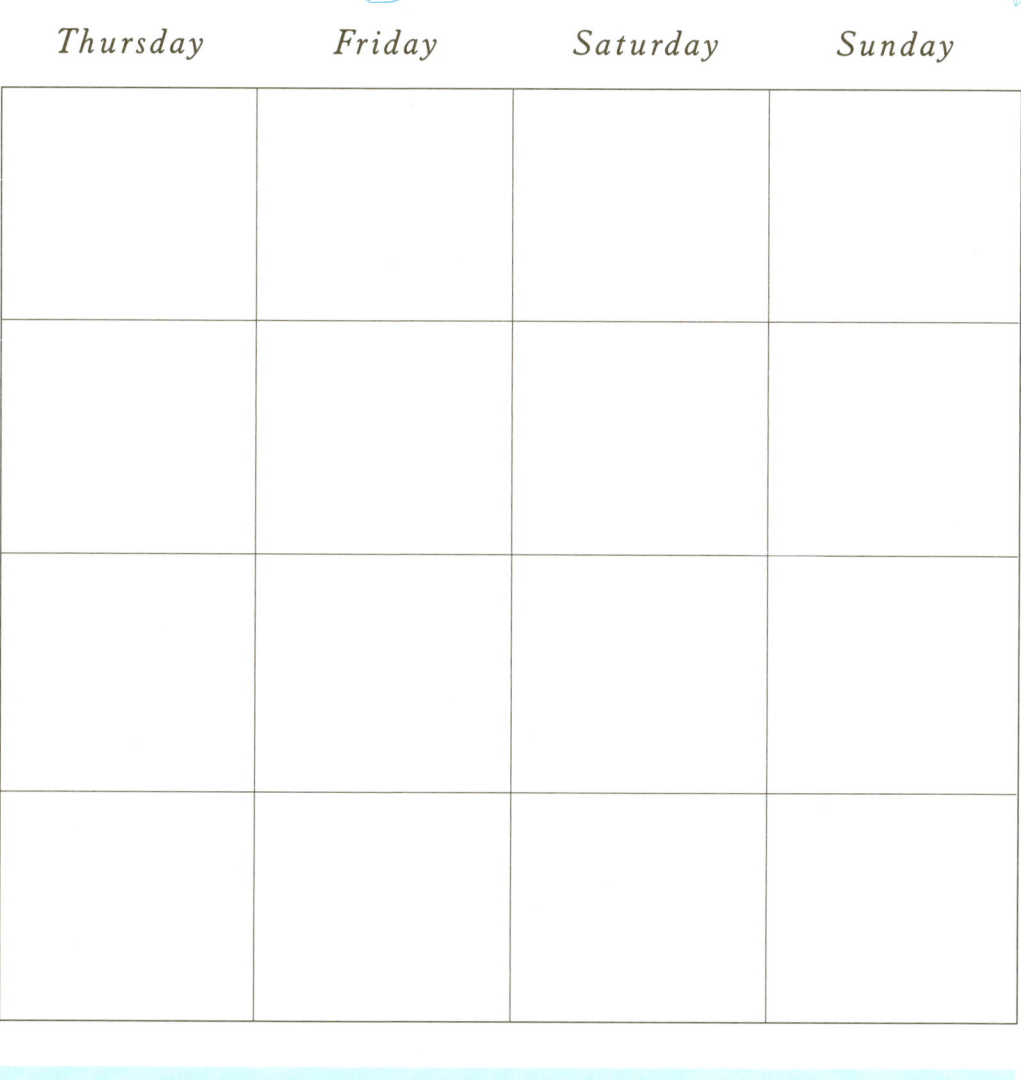

Thursday	Friday	Saturday	Sunday

REFLECTIONS

JOY TO EMBRACE	STRESS TO RELEASE	FOCUSING ON	GRATITUDE FOR

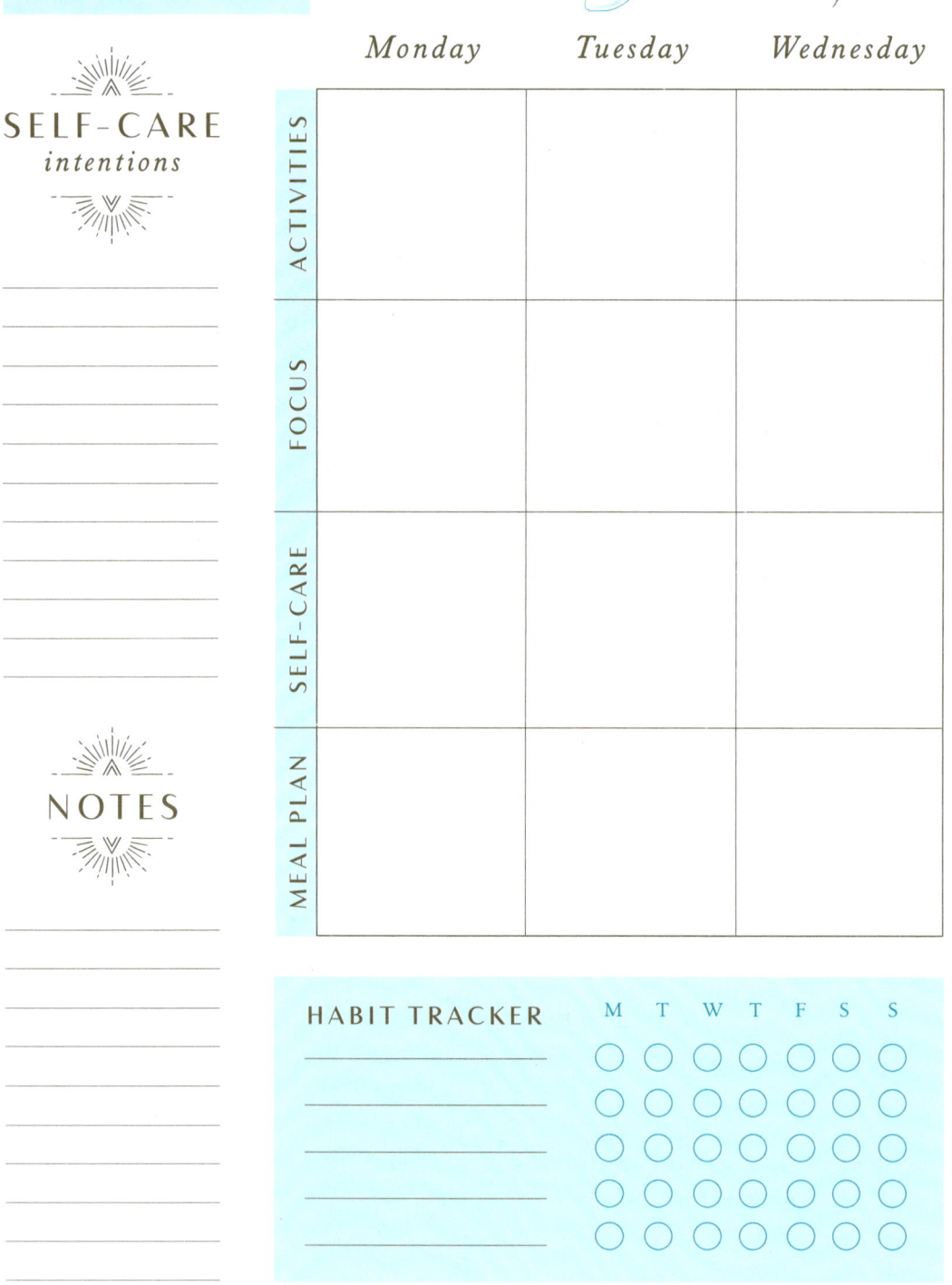

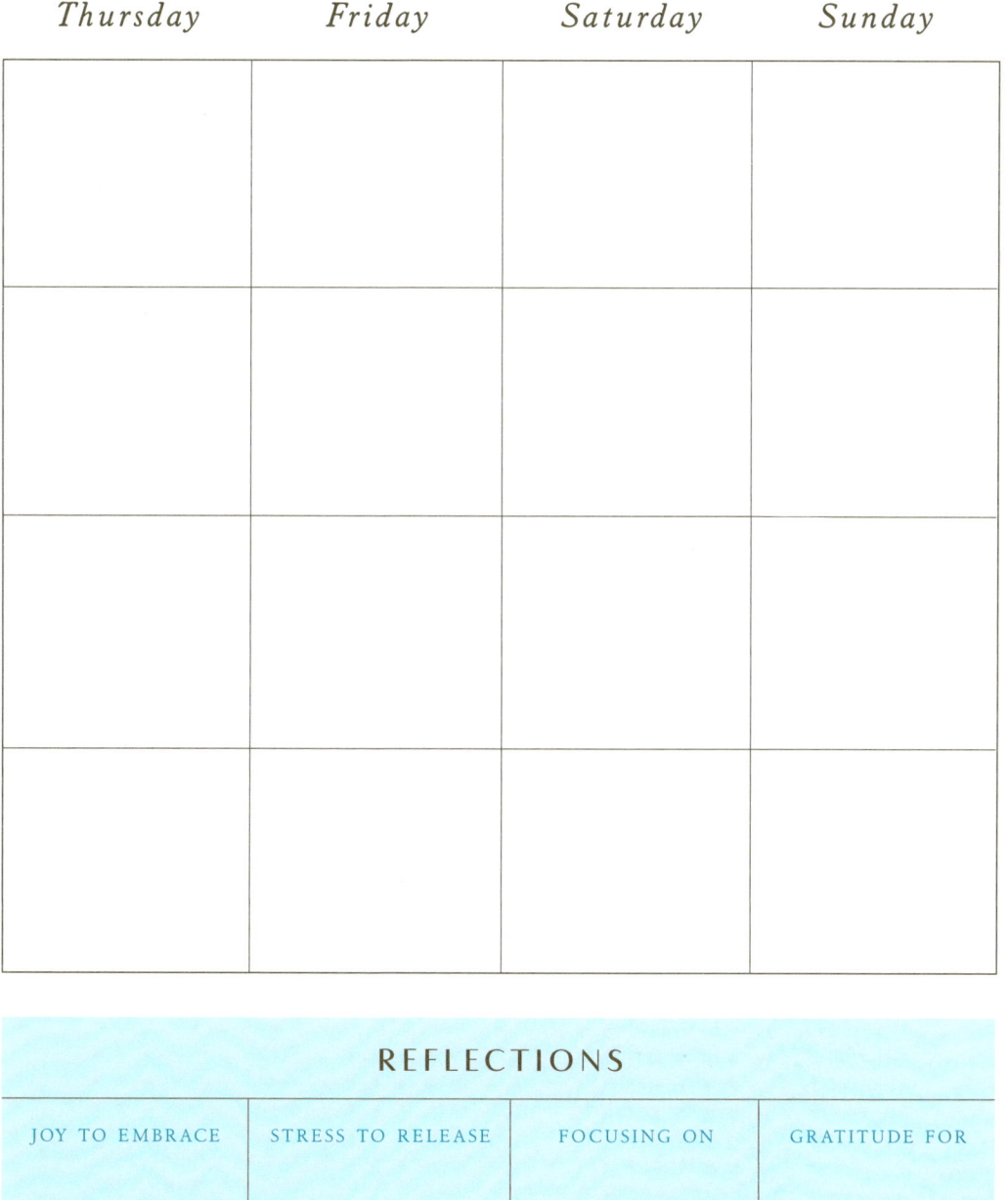

Thursday	Friday	Saturday	Sunday

REFLECTIONS

JOY TO EMBRACE	STRESS TO RELEASE	FOCUSING ON	GRATITUDE FOR

SELF-CARE
intentions

NOTES

	Monday	Tuesday	Wednesday
ACTIVITIES			
FOCUS			
SELF-CARE			
MEAL PLAN			

HABIT TRACKER

M T W T F S S

Thursday	Friday	Saturday	Sunday

REFLECTIONS

JOY TO EMBRACE	STRESS TO RELEASE	FOCUSING ON	GRATITUDE FOR

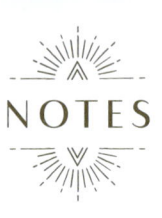

NOTES

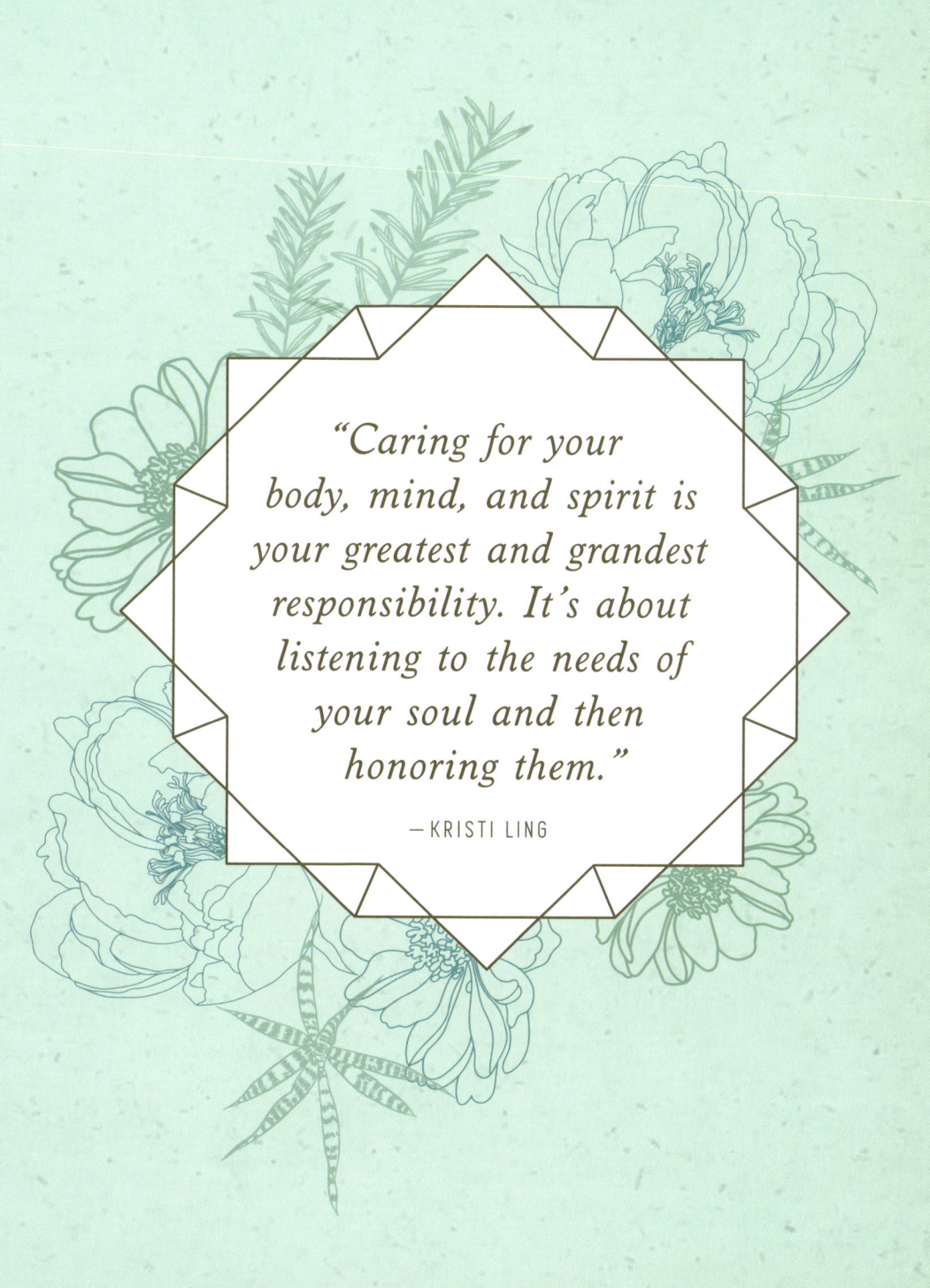

"Caring for your body, mind, and spirit is your greatest and grandest responsibility. It's about listening to the needs of your soul and then honoring them."

—KRISTI LING

SELF-CARE *priorities*

	Monday	Tuesday	Wednesday

IT IS A STRENGTH TO LAUGH AND TO ABANDON ONESELF, TO BE LIGHT.
—*Frida Kahlo*

NOTES

Thursday	Friday	Saturday	Sunday

BIRTHDAYS

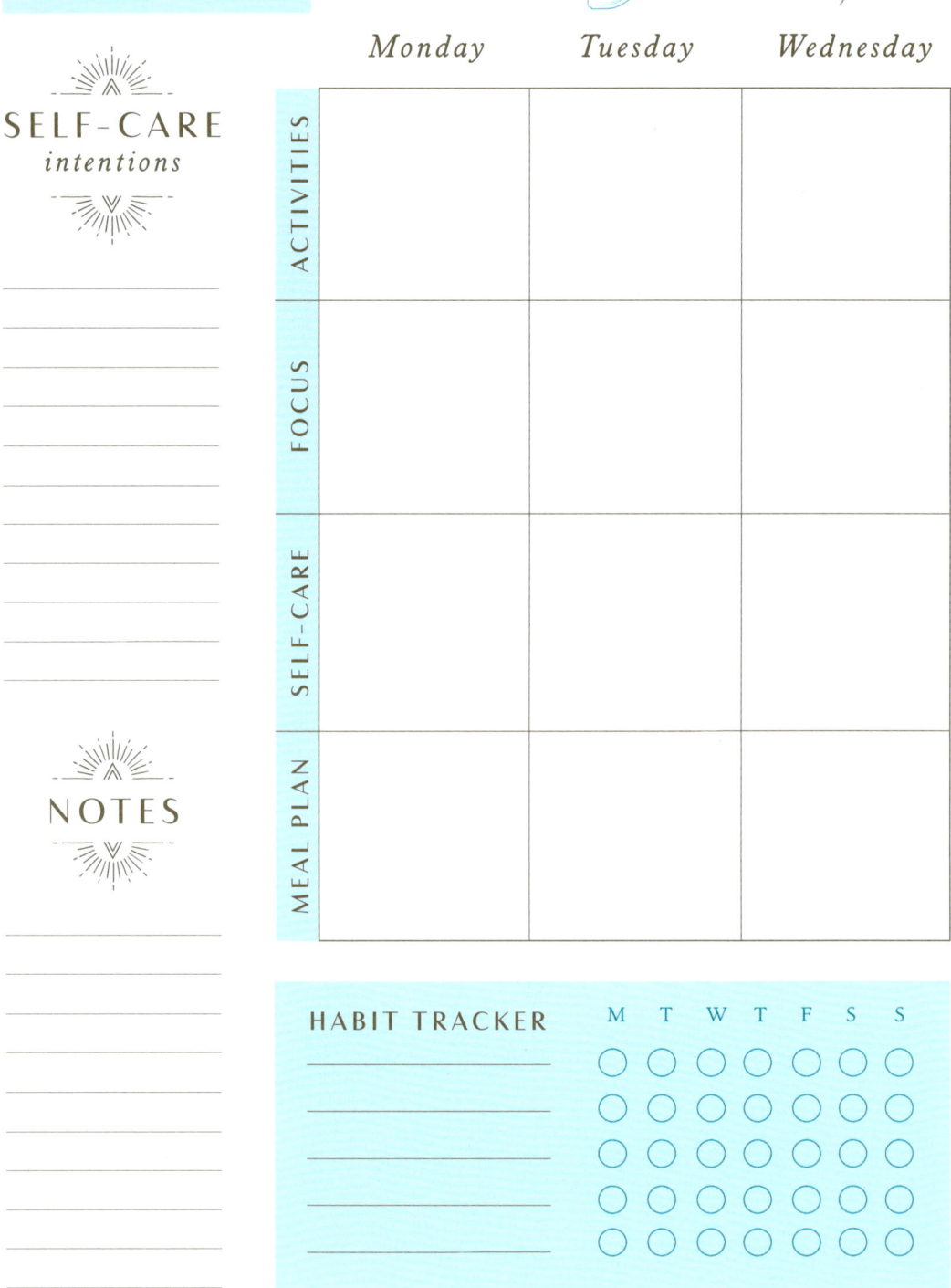

Thursday	Friday	Saturday	Sunday

REFLECTIONS

JOY TO EMBRACE	STRESS TO RELEASE	FOCUSING ON	GRATITUDE FOR

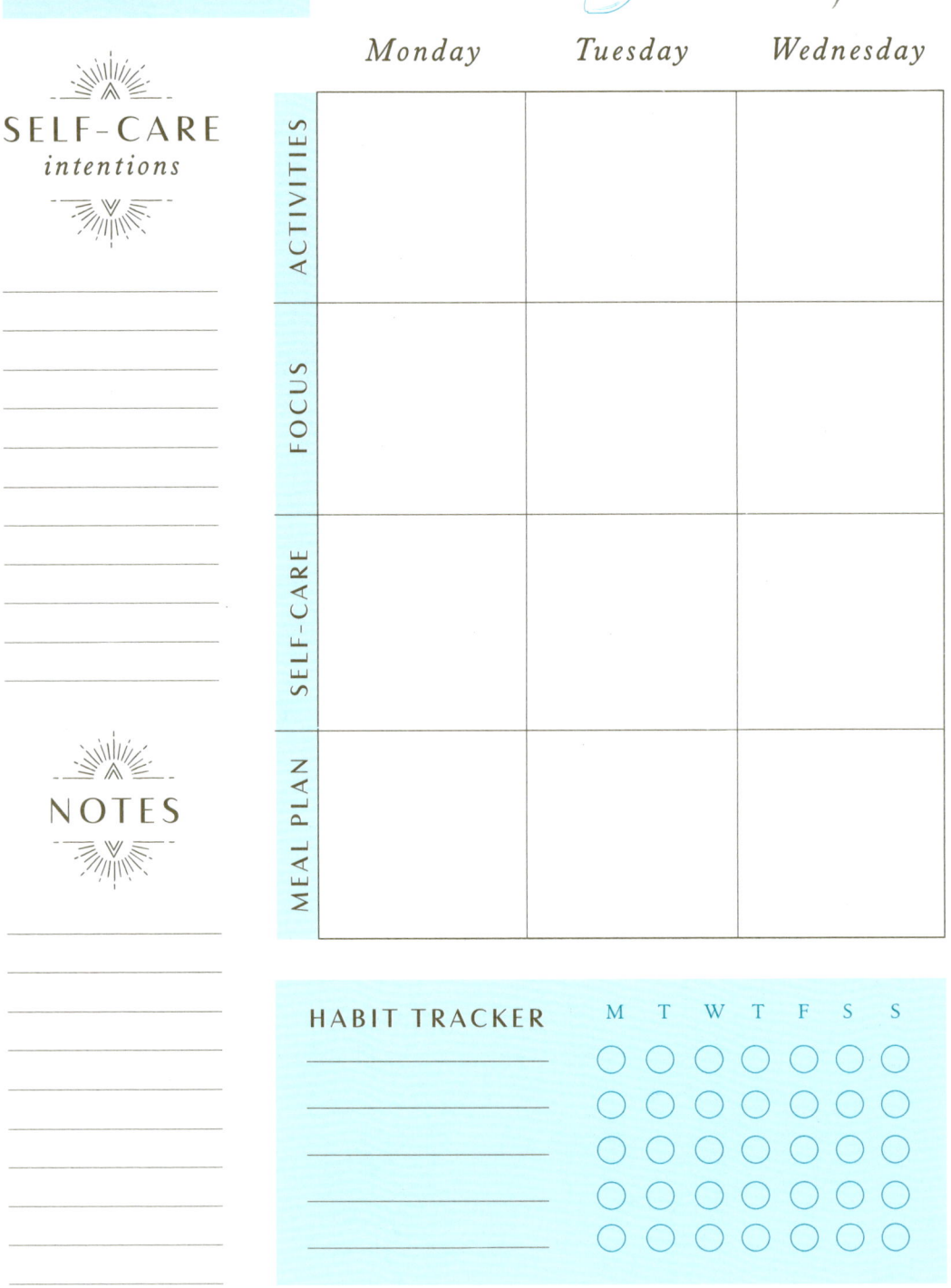

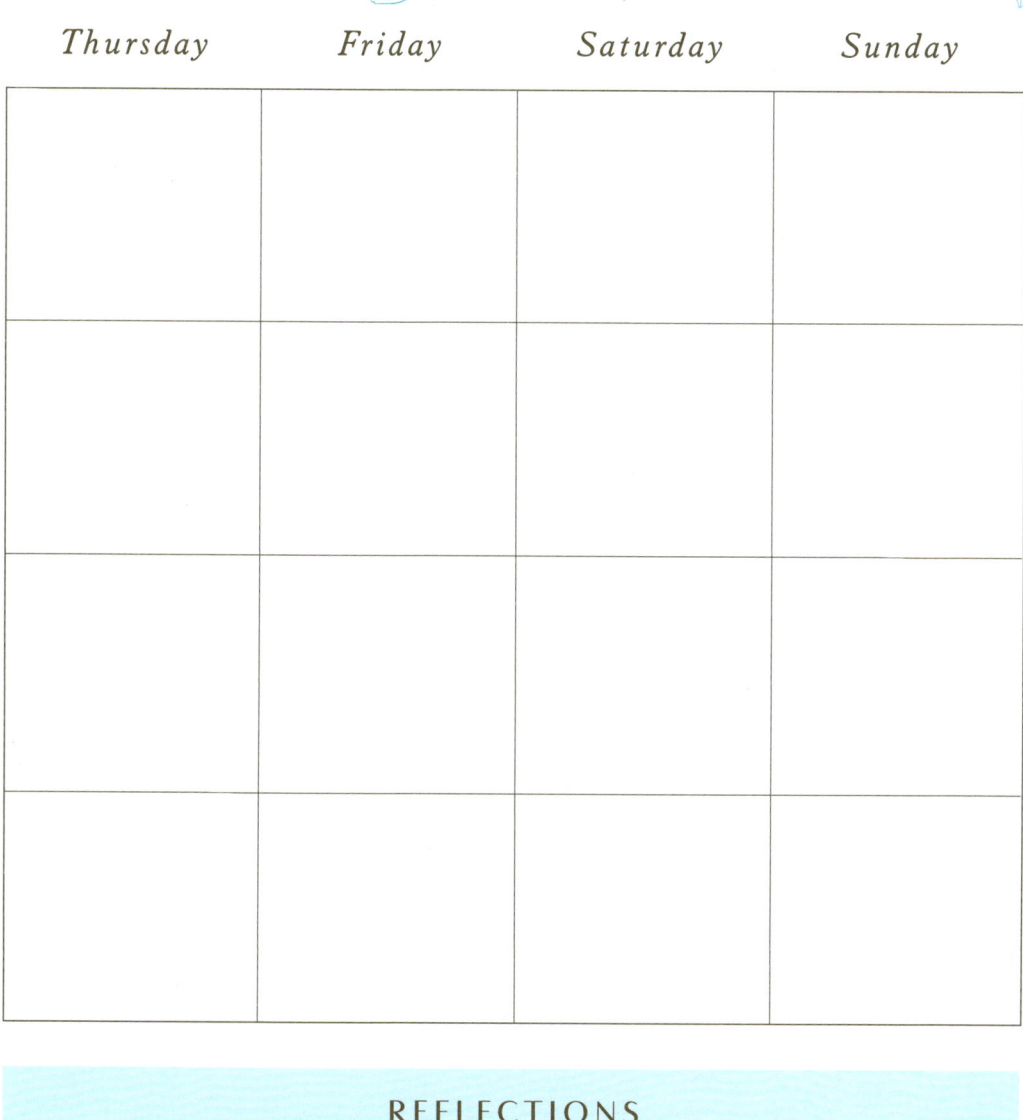

Thursday	Friday	Saturday	Sunday

REFLECTIONS

JOY TO EMBRACE	STRESS TO RELEASE	FOCUSING ON	GRATITUDE FOR

SELF-CARE
intentions

	Monday	Tuesday	Wednesday
ACTIVITIES			
FOCUS			
SELF-CARE			
MEAL PLAN			

NOTES

HABIT TRACKER

M T W T F S S

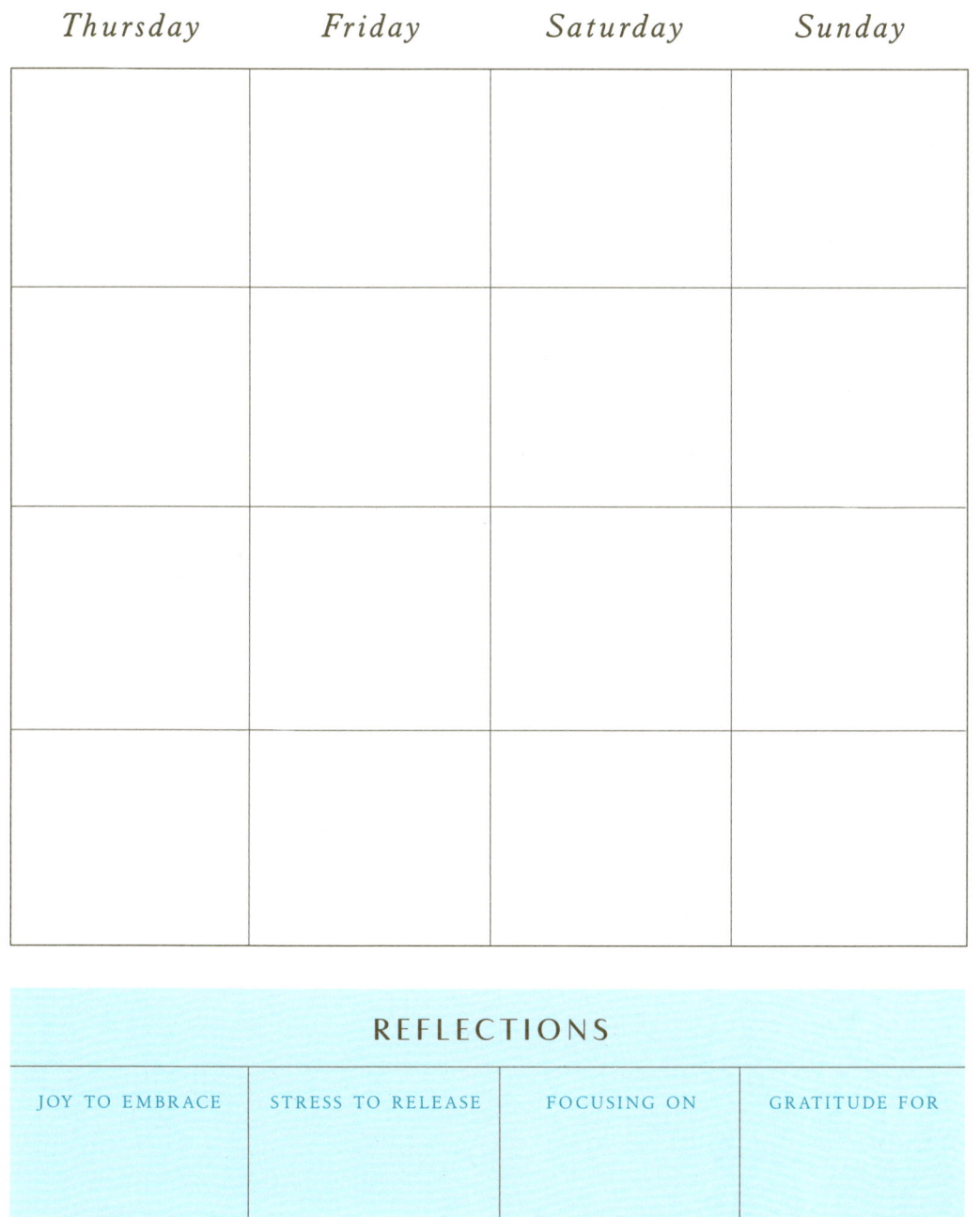

Thursday	Friday	Saturday	Sunday

REFLECTIONS

JOY TO EMBRACE	STRESS TO RELEASE	FOCUSING ON	GRATITUDE FOR

SELF-CARE
intentions

	Monday	Tuesday	Wednesday
ACTIVITIES			
FOCUS			
SELF-CARE			
MEAL PLAN			

NOTES

HABIT TRACKER

	M	T	W	T	F	S	S
___	○	○	○	○	○	○	○
___	○	○	○	○	○	○	○
___	○	○	○	○	○	○	○
___	○	○	○	○	○	○	○
___	○	○	○	○	○	○	○

Thursday	Friday	Saturday	Sunday

REFLECTIONS

JOY TO EMBRACE	STRESS TO RELEASE	FOCUSING ON	GRATITUDE FOR

SELF-CARE *intentions*

	Monday	Tuesday	Wednesday
ACTIVITIES			
FOCUS			
SELF-CARE			
MEAL PLAN			

NOTES

HABIT TRACKER

	M	T	W	T	F	S	S
	○	○	○	○	○	○	○
	○	○	○	○	○	○	○
	○	○	○	○	○	○	○
	○	○	○	○	○	○	○
	○	○	○	○	○	○	○

Thursday	Friday	Saturday	Sunday

REFLECTIONS

JOY TO EMBRACE	STRESS TO RELEASE	FOCUSING ON	GRATITUDE FOR

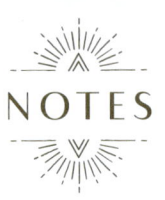

NOTES

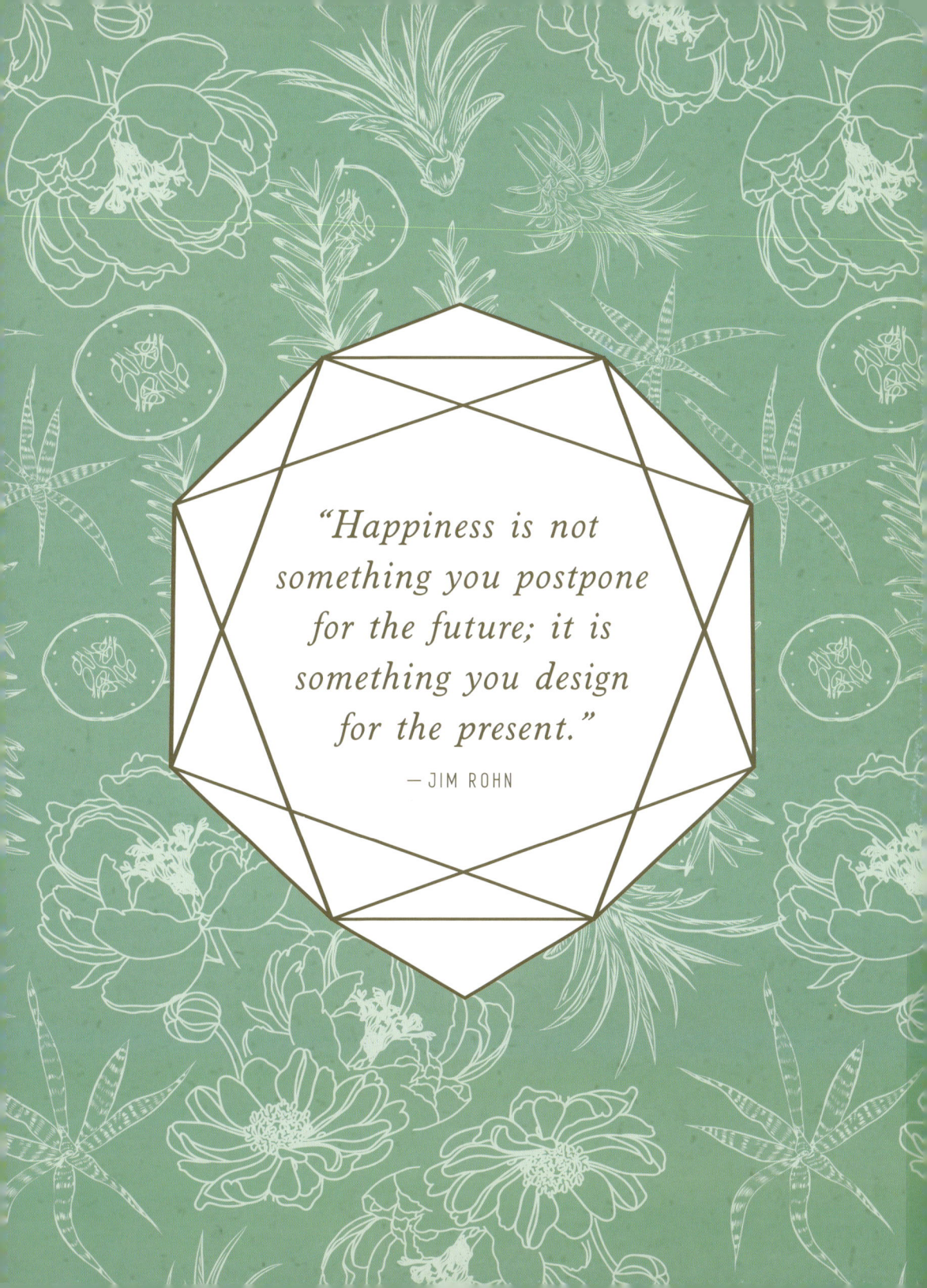

"Happiness is not something you postpone for the future; it is something you design for the present."

— JIM ROHN

SELF-CARE *priorities*

	Monday	Tuesday	Wednesday

LEARN TO VALUE YOURSELF, WHICH MEANS: FIGHT FOR YOUR HAPPINESS.
—Ayn Rand

NOTES

Thursday	Friday	Saturday	Sunday

BIRTHDAYS

SELF-CARE
intentions

	Monday	Tuesday	Wednesday
ACTIVITIES			
FOCUS			
SELF-CARE			
MEAL PLAN			

NOTES

HABIT TRACKER

	M	T	W	T	F	S	S
_____	○	○	○	○	○	○	○
_____	○	○	○	○	○	○	○
_____	○	○	○	○	○	○	○
_____	○	○	○	○	○	○	○
_____	○	○	○	○	○	○	○

Thursday	Friday	Saturday	Sunday

REFLECTIONS

JOY TO EMBRACE	STRESS TO RELEASE	FOCUSING ON	GRATITUDE FOR

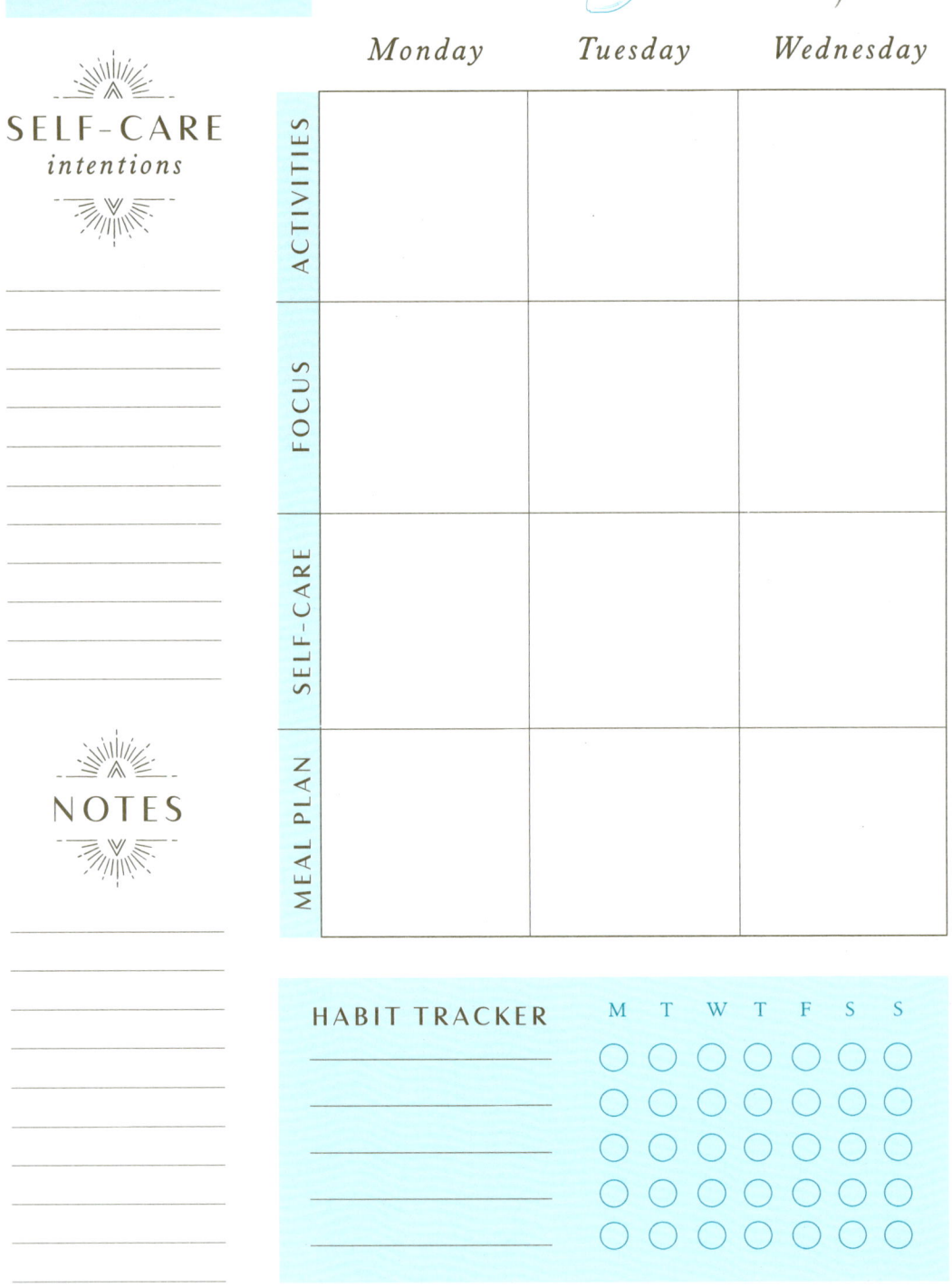

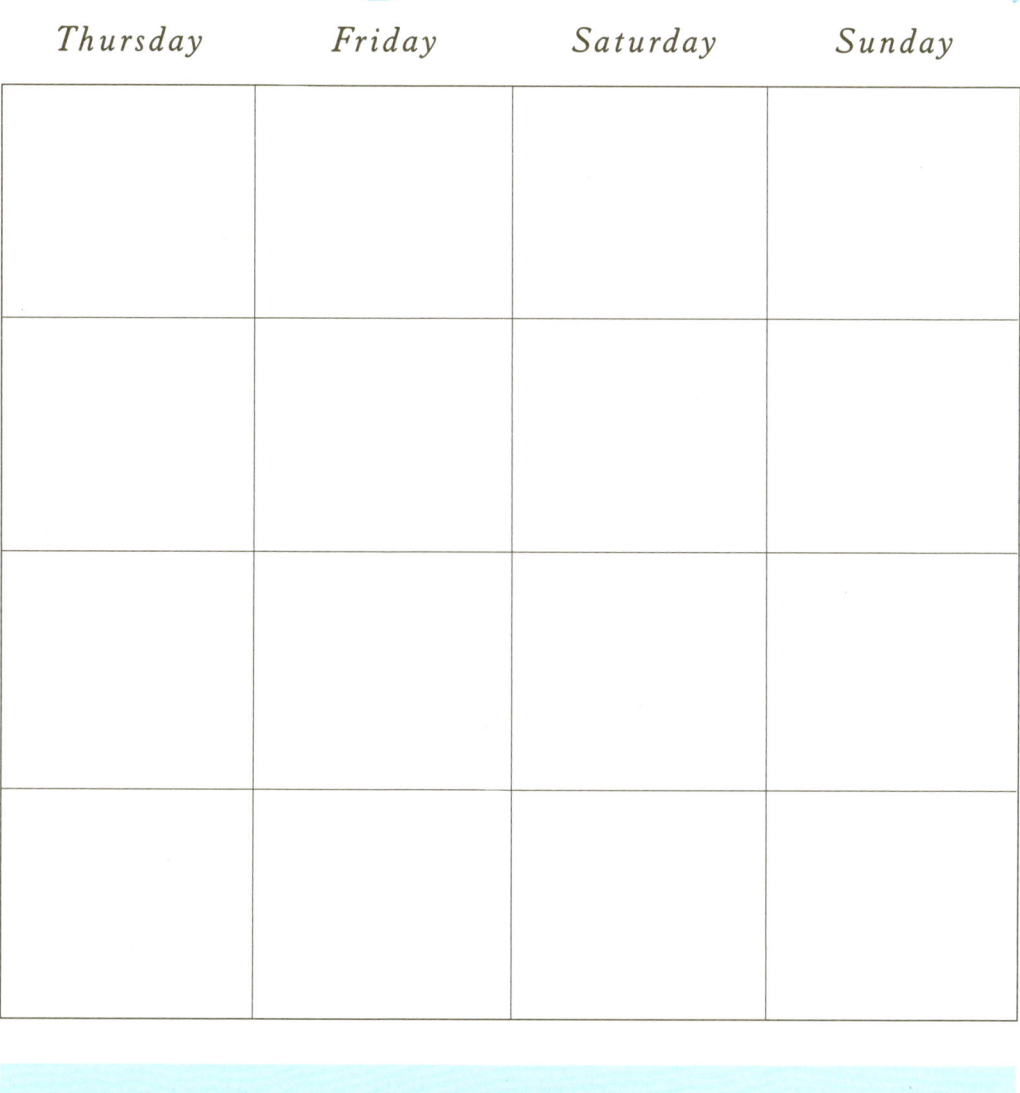

Thursday	Friday	Saturday	Sunday

REFLECTIONS

JOY TO EMBRACE	STRESS TO RELEASE	FOCUSING ON	GRATITUDE FOR

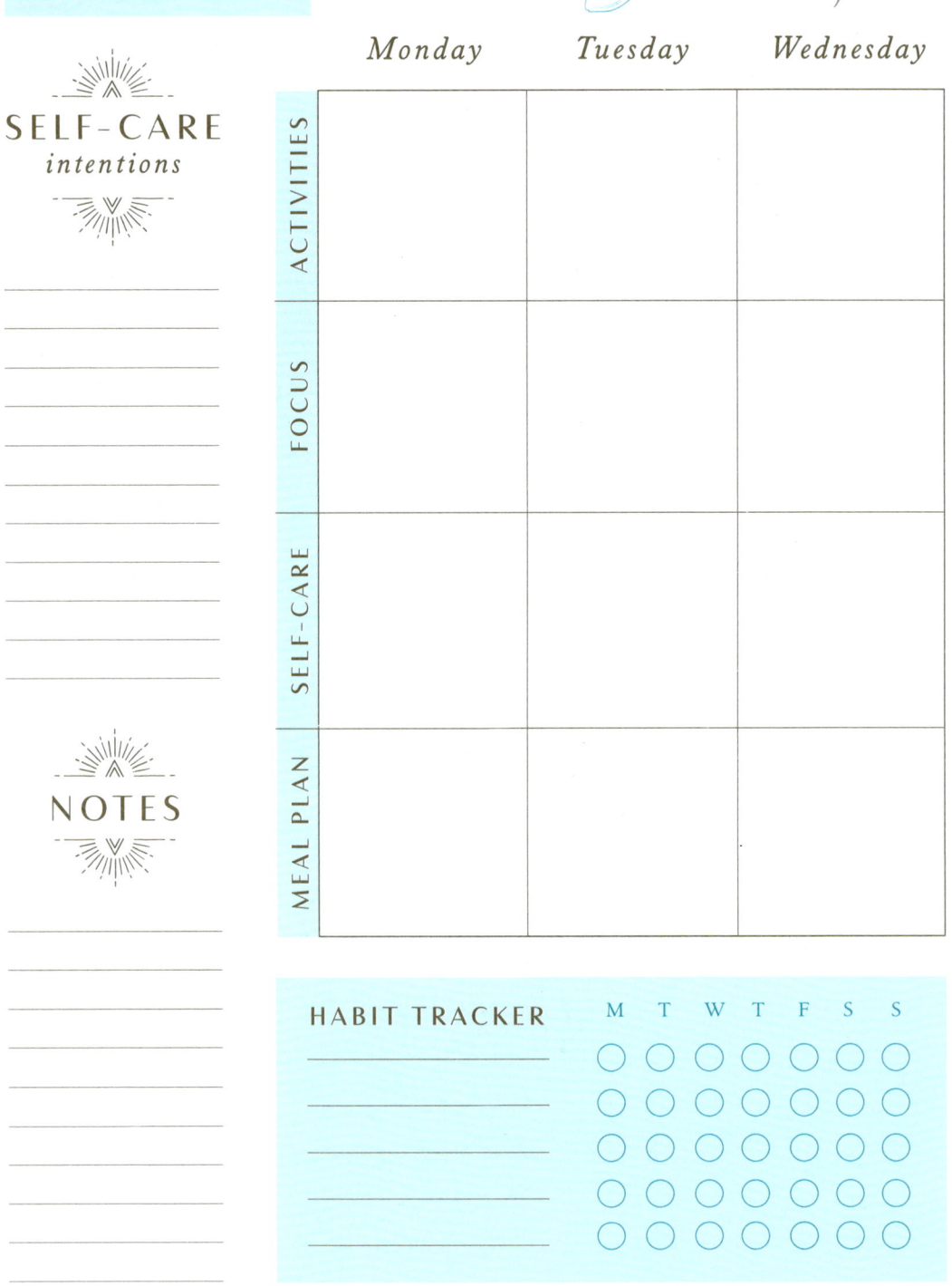

Thursday	Friday	Saturday	Sunday

REFLECTIONS

JOY TO EMBRACE	STRESS TO RELEASE	FOCUSING ON	GRATITUDE FOR

SELF-CARE
intentions

	Monday	Tuesday	Wednesday
ACTIVITIES			
FOCUS			
SELF-CARE			
MEAL PLAN			

NOTES

HABIT TRACKER

	M	T	W	T	F	S	S
_____	○	○	○	○	○	○	○
_____	○	○	○	○	○	○	○
_____	○	○	○	○	○	○	○
_____	○	○	○	○	○	○	○
_____	○	○	○	○	○	○	○

Thursday	Friday	Saturday	Sunday

REFLECTIONS

JOY TO EMBRACE	STRESS TO RELEASE	FOCUSING ON	GRATITUDE FOR

SELF-CARE
intentions

	Monday	Tuesday	Wednesday
ACTIVITIES			
FOCUS			
SELF-CARE			
MEAL PLAN			

NOTES

HABIT TRACKER

	M	T	W	T	F	S	S
	○	○	○	○	○	○	○
	○	○	○	○	○	○	○
	○	○	○	○	○	○	○
	○	○	○	○	○	○	○
	○	○	○	○	○	○	○

Thursday	Friday	Saturday	Sunday

REFLECTIONS

JOY TO EMBRACE	STRESS TO RELEASE	FOCUSING ON	GRATITUDE FOR

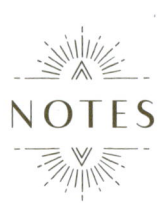

NOTES

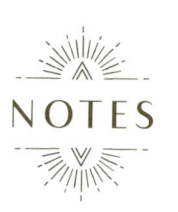
NOTES

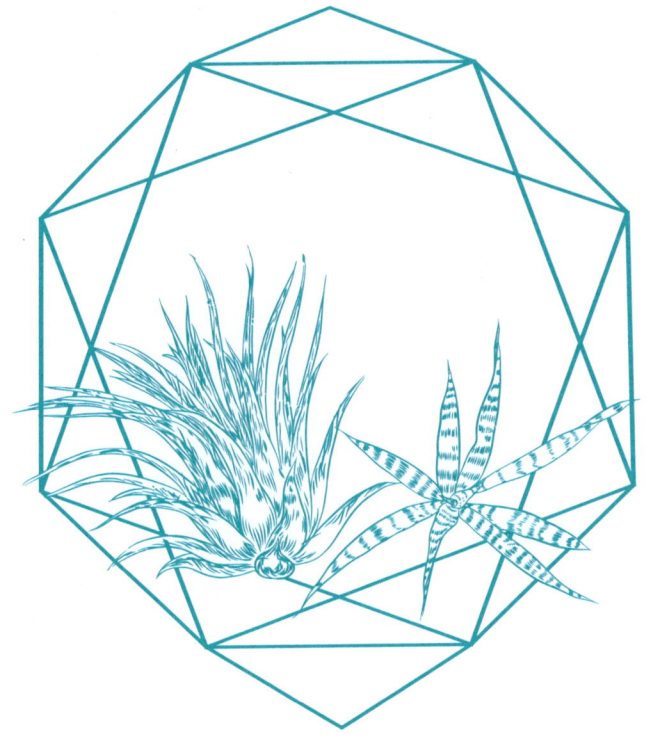

INSIGHTS

an imprint of

INSIGHT EDITIONS

www.insighteditions.com

Copyright © 2021 Insight Editions.
All rights reserved.

MANUFACTURED IN CHINA

10 9 8 7 6 5 4 3 2 1